Praise f___
of Your Ch

"This dan(.y pocket-sized book is packed with sensible tips for preparing children (and their parents) for outpatient, short-stay, or long-term hospitalization. Sidebars offer real-life suggestions from parents who've 'been there, done that.'"

ial

DUE

"When you are p___ __ __ up the stuffed animals and pajam__ ___ ___ to the hospital, make sure t.__ take this book with you. Chock full of informa..on about how to deal with testing, f.nances, siblings and schoolwork, this guide is handy and easy to read."

— *Atlanta Constitution*

• • • • •

"*Your Child in the Hospital is a practical book of tips and wisdom from veteran parents that will help make any hospital stay easier.* "

— *Library Journal*, Nursing Your Children's Health Collection

• • • • •

"When your child is ill or injured, the hospital setting can be overwhelming. Here is a terrific roadmap to help keep families on track."

— James B. Fahner, MD
Division Chief, DeVos Children's Hospital
Grand Rapids, MI

• • • • •

"This revised edition of a popular book contains simple, no nonsense advice on how to make hospitalizations easier for the whole family, whether a child is going to the hospital for stitches, outpatient surgery, or a longer stay."

— *Our Children, The National PTA Magazine*

• • • • •

"In clear, easy-to-read text, this book provides valuable tips to assist both child and parent in coping with any hospital encounter. An excellent resource."

— Oncology Nursing Society

"This is a straightforward, useful book for anyone whose child is facing long-term or short-term hospitalization."

— Parents' Press

"Written with sensitivity and common sense born of experience and knowledge, it offers solid, practical advice."

— Journal of Child-Care Administration

"For a parent, taking a child to the hospital and facing the uncertainties ahead can also be scary. Your Child in the Hospital is designed to make that time in the hospital a little easier for children and their parents."

— Pittsburgh Post-Gazette

"When their children are in the hospital, panicky parents need support—someone with helping hands and a caring heart. Helpful guidelines are offered in Your Child in the Hospital."

— Nashville Tennessean

"An excellent resource for any parent whose child must be hospitalized. It contains information on preparation for hospital visits, brief procedures and long-term illnesses. Stories from parents give first hand advice."

— L.A. Parent

"The practice of pediatrics not only must remember to address children's fears but also should help parents to do the same. In a what-to-expect manner, this parent-centered guide offers concrete, useful insights into how hospitals function and how parents can comfortably become part of the process."

— Laura A. Jana, MD
Co-Founder, The Dr. Spock Company

Your Child in the Hospital

the Hospital

A Practical Guide for Parents

Third Edition

Nancy Keene

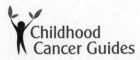

Childhood
Cancer Guides

Your Child in the Hospital: A Practical Guide for Parents, Third Edition

by Nancy Keene

Copyright © 2015 Childhood Cancer Guides

Published by Childhood Cancer Guides, P.O. Box 31937, Bellingham, WA 98228
Printed in the United States of America

362.1108

Keene

Printing History:
1997: First Edition
1999: Second Edition

For information about special discounts for bulk purchases, please contact Independent Publishers Group Special Sales at specialmarkets@ipgbook.com.

ISBN 978-1-941089-99-6

Library of Congress Control Number: 2014919823

To my daughters
Kathryn and Alison

Contents

Introduction

WHY DO I HAVE TO GO TO THE HOSPITAL? Will they hurt me? Are you going to leave me there? How long will I stay? These are some of the questions your child might ask before a trip to the hospital. Hospitals are fascinating, but sometimes frightening, places for children. They are full of beds with bars, buzzing machinery, and unfamiliar adults. Your child may be sick or hurt when she first enters this strange, new place. She may also be very worried.

For a parent, taking a child to the hospital can be scary as well. You must put your child in someone else's hands and you may worry that there is no way to ease your child's fears. However, you can do plenty to prepare your child both physically and emotionally for a stay in the hospital. You can learn about your child's illness or injury and answer his questions honestly. You can work in partnership with the medical team to give your child the very best that modern medicine has to offer. You can pack a favorite teddy bear, book, or game. All of these actions will help your child feel safe and comfortable.

If you know what to expect once you and your child get to the hospital, you can make hospital routines more predictable, and even fun. Tips on taking pills, having x-rays, and dealing with IVs can help make these procedures easier to manage. Decorating the hospital room and visiting child life specialists will make your child's stay more cheerful, and forming a close working relationship with your child's doctors and nurses will increase your entire family's peace of mind. Knowing what to expect will help ease your fears and empower you to be a strong advocate for your child.

Being your child's advocate may be a new role for you. This book will help you work more effectively with medical personnel by discussing how to:

- **Make a plan.** Consider what to bring to the hospital, how to prepare your child for her stay, and ways to adjust your work schedule and deal with your child's schooling.

- **Educate yourself.** Learn about the treatment, surgery, doctor, and hospital, and how to find materials to help prepare your child.

- **Communicate.** Work with family members, doctors, and nurses to build a team that will focus on your child's care. Help to ensure that your child's doctor hears your concerns and that you understand the doctor.

- **Be a role model.** Learn how other parents comforted their children and coped with their children's behavior changes during and after the trip to the hospital.

This book also covers topics such as helpful things your family members and friends can do and say while your child is in the hospital, and how you can include brothers and sisters before and during the hospitalization. If your child is in the hospital for weeks or months, you'll find tips on how to work with the school so your child will not get too far behind. In addition, all parents of hospitalized children need to manage insurance, bills, and medical records, so those topics are covered as well.

In addition, stories from more than forty parents describe their children's hospitalizations and offer advice to help you prepare. These parents share how they answered their children's questions, cleared up misconceptions, and got them ready to go. Their stories show how good preparation transformed their children's fears into curiosity and cooperation. However, every family is unique. Your child's hospital visit may be a whirlwind affair, but other children may be in the hospital for months. Because each family has different needs, this book presents a range of suggestions and stories. You will be able to pick the tips that will best help your child. Don't expect to follow the advice of all forty parents—that might become overwhelming rather than empowering. Instead, think of the book as a rich menu of choices.

This book covers emergency room visits, short-term stays, and lengthy hospitalizations. It contains journal pages where children can express their feelings about their hospitalization through words or drawings. A packing list will help you decide what to bring along.

At the end of the book is a *Resources* section that lists books for parents and children of all ages. Organizations that help families with hospitalizations are also included.

Because both boys and girls are hospitalized, we did not use only masculine personal pronouns (he, him). Instead, we alternated pronouns (e.g., she, he) within chapters. This may seem awkward as you read, but it prevents half of the parents who read the book from feeling that the text does not apply to their child.

You know your child best. That knowledge, the information in this book, and the advice from forty parents who have been there, will help your family cope with your child's hospitalization.

❦

Best wishes for a positive hospital experience for you, your child, and your entire family. May your child be prepared well, treated with warmth and kindness, healed of the illness or injury, and home soon.

Chapter 1

Before You Go

*"Never look back unless you
are planning to go that way."*

— Henry David Thoreau

MOST PARENTS WOULD BE GLAD never to have to take their child to the hospital. Hospitals can be noisy, overwhelming, frightening places for children as well as parents. However, being prepared and getting the information you need before taking your child to the hospital can make the experience much easier for you, your child, and the rest of your family.

Is hospitalization necessary?

In emergencies, you may not have time to ask the doctor questions about your child's hospitalization. But, in most circumstances, you can discuss the reasons for hospitalization with your child's doctor in advance. Here are a few important questions to ask when your child's doctor recommends hospitalization:

* Why is hospitalization necessary?

* Which hospital is best for my child?

* Are there any alternatives such as outpatient surgery?

* Who will perform the procedure or surgery?

* Would you explain the procedure or surgery in detail and in language that I understand?

* Are books, pamphlets, or videos available that describe the procedure or surgery?

* Is there a child life specialist on staff who will discuss the hospitalization with my child and answer his questions in advance?

* Will our insurance cover it?

Try to get enough information to help you and your child prepare for medical treatments and procedures. Knowing what to expect will lower your anxiety level as well as your child's.

> When Claire had her tonsils out, they did it as an outpatient surgery. At first I was shocked that they were going to send my daughter home after just a few hours, but now I'm so glad they did. I think it's almost always better to be at home if you can be. It's more cost effective and your child can benefit from a familiar environment and the comforts of home.

Get a second opinion

Most doctors welcome consultations and encourage second opinions. There are many gray areas in medicine where judgment and experience are as important as knowledge. In addition, many insurance companies require a second opinion. If, after discussions with the doctor, you are still uneasy about any aspect of your child's medical care, do not hesitate to seek another opinion.

There are two ways to get a second opinion: see another specialist, or ask your child's doctor to arrange a multidisciplinary second opinion. Many parents get a second opinion before moving ahead with any but the most routine or emergency treatment. You do not need to do this in secret. Explain to your child's doctor that, before proceeding, you would like a second opinion.

Try to find an independent doctor to provide the second opinion because it may be tough for doctors who share a practice or regularly give each other referrals to provide entirely objective opinions. To allow for a thorough analysis, arrange to have copies of all records sent ahead to the doctor who will give the second opinion.

Sometimes, with complex illnesses or injuries, a group of specialists will meet to review the case. Ask your doctor about this type of multidisciplinary review if you believe your child needs one.

Parents often hesitate to ask for a second opinion because they are afraid of offending their child's doctor. Your child's doctor should not resent it if you seek a second opinion. If she does resist, explain that you need a second opinion to feel comfortable proceeding with the proposed treatment.

> *When Ian's doctor recommended surgery to correct his eyes, which were starting to turn in, I was very reluctant to agree because Ian was so young. The doctor told me that without surgery, his eyes could get worse and would not be able to be treated in the future. I talked to a lot of other people and got a second opinion. At that point, we felt much more comfortable going ahead with the surgery.*

Find a specialist

Often a hospitalized child will need a specialist to perform surgery, give anesthesia, or provide other treatment. Your choice of specialists may be limited by the hospital, location, time constraints, or insurance restrictions. Usually, your child's pediatrician will recommend an appropriate specialist (e.g., a pediatric surgeon). Make sure that your insurance will cover the specialist you choose.

The following list may help you feel more comfortable with the recommended specialist. If you have time, make sure that your child's specialist:

• Is board-certified. This means that the doctor has passed rigorous written and oral tests given by a board of examiners in his or her specialty. You can call the American Board of Medical Specialties at (866) ASK-ABMS (275-2267) or visit *https://www. certificationmatters.org/is-your-doctor-board-certified/search-now.aspx* to find out if your child's specialist is board certified.

• Establishes a good rapport with your child

• Communicates clearly and compassionately

• Answers all questions in a way that is easy to understand

• Consults with other doctors about complex problems

• Makes all test results available

• Is willing to let you participate in the decision-making process

• Respects your values

Often the specialist your child's doctor recommends is a good match and the family finds him easy to communicate with, competent, and caring. If you don't develop a good rapport with the first specialist recommended to you, ask for or locate another doctor.

> We had a wonderful relationship with the specialist at the children's hospital. He perfectly blended the science and art of medicine. His manner was warm, he was extremely qualified professionally, and he was very easy to talk with. He welcomed discussions with us about our daughter's treatment. Although he was busy, we never felt rushed. I laughed when I saw that he had written in the chart, "Mother asks innumerable appropriate questions."

Make a plan

Begin planning your child's hospitalization as soon as you find out that it is necessary. Even a brief hospital stay can be physically draining and emotionally difficult, so take time before the visit to prepare your child and the rest of your family.

- Arrange care for your other children. This should be with someone they know and like who can help the siblings carry on with their normal routine (school, music lessons, sports). Also, child care should be flexible in case you need to stay longer than planned at the hospital.

- Plan how you will keep your household functioning. Find a friend or neighbor to feed animals, water the plants, and pick up mail.

- Take time off work and notify your child's school. If the hospitalization might be lengthy, read Chapter 15 for ways to work with your child's school.

- Make a list of the names and telephone numbers of people you can call on for help. Consider designating one person to call family members and friends to share news, coordinate food, or baby-sit.

- Pack ahead of time. Your child might want to help choose which clothes, toys, and books to take to the hospital. You can use the *Packing List* in the back of this book to figure out what to bring.

- Plan how you will prepare your child and her siblings for the visit. Consider whether your child might be comforted by a hospital tour, a talk with the doctor, or a chat with other children who have undergone similar treatment. You might visit your local library or the hospital library to find books about your child's illness or injury or about hospital stays. The *Resources* section in the back of this book contains suggested reading.

> *My daughter has been hospitalized twice to control her seizures. To prepare, I went to the library and took out every book they had on seizure disorders. I asked the neurologist if he had any books to recommend. Then I went to the school nurse and asked her to give other parents of children who had seizures my name and telephone number. I contacted the Epilepsy Foundation and they sent loads of literature plus a list of people to contact. Talking to the other parents and reading books really helped us plan for hospitalizations.*

Chapter 2

The Emergency Room

"The best way out is always through."
— Robert Frost

DOCTORS AND NURSES IN EMERGENCY ROOMS treat serious trauma and illnesses every day. They work under stressful conditions and may not have time to explain what is going on or make your visit comfortable. Often, especially on Friday and Saturday nights, the emergency room is full. During very busy times, you'll probably wait for a long time if your child's condition isn't life-threatening.

Avoid the emergency room if possible

Try to avoid the emergency room whenever possible. Your child's pediatrician or a walk-in clinic often will treat your child more quickly and efficiently than an emergency room. In addition, the pediatrician is more familiar with your child and less expensive than the emergency room.

Many parents also try to avoid taking their child to the hospital in an ambulance. In some areas, public ambulance service is free; in other regions, the shortest of ambulance rides can cost hundreds of dollars. However, do not drive if the emergency is life-threatening, if your child may require treatment during transport, or if you are too worried to drive safely. When in doubt, call an ambulance.

> When my teenaged daughter tore a ligament in her knee early one Saturday morning, we called our doctor, and he said to go to the emergency room to get a diagnosis and then call the orthopedic surgeon to make an appointment for further treatment and follow-up. We knew we might have to wait a long time, so we each brought a book and practiced being patient.

If you have time, call the pediatrician before you go to the emergency room. She may be able to suggest a treatment option that helps you avoid the emergency room altogether. If you must go, your child's pediatrician may be able to meet you there. In addition to a comforting presence, your child's doctor can provide a second opinion, a referral, or pertinent information about your child's medical history.

It can also help to bring your spouse or another adult who acts as an advocate while you comfort your child. The advocate can call family or employers, fill out paperwork, and ask questions. Having another adult present allows you to stay at your child's side so that you can attend to her needs.

Bring something to do

Emergency rooms pick the most urgent cases to treat first. Depending on the emergency room's patient load and your child's needs, you may wait hours for treatment.

> One evening my 3-year-old, Gylany, fell off the couch, hit her head on the floor, and passed out for a few seconds. I scooped her up, grabbed my 5-year-old, and went to the emergency room. We checked in, then waited for over 2 hours. My kids were exhausted from crying. Whenever I asked the receptionist how long it would be, she said, "They will be right with you." Gylany threw up, and we still waited a half hour before they finally saw us. We were there until one thirty in the morning.

Even if you have just a moment before bringing your child in, try to grab something to comfort and distract your child: a stuffed animal, a familiar book, some crayons, or a computer game. If you don't have time to bring something, ask at the emergency room desk. Many emergency rooms keep some toys on hand for such occasions.

You should also try to explain to your child what will happen during the visit. Even if you don't know the details, you can explain that the doctor will ask lots of questions, do an examination, and help her feel better. Reassure her that you will stay with her the whole time.

Stay with your child

Whenever your child goes to the emergency room, he should have a reassuring parent present if possible. At times, staff members may try to keep you out of treatment areas. Doctors and nurses might worry that you will get in their way or further agitate your child. If you are very emotional, these may be valid concerns. However, you usually can insist on staying with your child if you are calm. Use your judgment—if your child is unconscious or has suffered severe trauma—it may be best to wait outside.

Most injuries and illnesses are not severe, and your child will probably draw more comfort from having you present than anyone else. You can provide great reassurance by holding your child's hand, singing, or quietly explaining what's happening.

> While the doctor manipulated the broken bone, I kept bodily contact with Aurora. I stroked what I could. At one point, I held her foot. It helped her be calm and feel connected. I stood at her foot when they were working by her head. I stayed where they weren't.

When you arrive in an emergency room, you must fill out paperwork, including medical history and insurance information. This can be time-consuming and, if your child is seriously ill or injured, hospital staff will want to begin treatment immediately. You can ask your spouse or a friend to handle the paperwork, or take it into the exam room.

Work with the staff

It's a good idea to establish rapport with emergency room staff right away. That means staying calm, providing accurate information, and gently but regularly making them aware of your presence. Prior to giving permission for medications, make sure you tell the doctor or nurse about any prescription or over-the-counter drugs that your child takes, for example, an asthma inhaler or an antihistamine.

Politely ask the doctors what they are doing and why. Try to understand the treatment plan for your child's illness or injury. If you are uneasy about the proposed treatment, ask for another opinion. In large teaching hospitals, the first doctor you see usually is a resident. Ask to see a chief resident or attending physician if you feel another opinion is necessary (the different types of doctors in teaching hospitals are explained in Chapter 5, *The Staff*).

> *One night, we took our 18-month-old daughter, who has diabetes, to the emergency room because of a sudden, severe ear infection. I had already checked her blood sugar and it was fine. But when they heard "diabetes," they immediately began to draw blood and put a urine bag on her. I said, "Stop for a moment and listen to me." After I explained, they just dealt with the infection.*

If your child will be going home with you, ask for all instructions in writing—you may not remember later. You might also ask about:

- Possible complications related to medication
- Side effects, such as swelling or fevers, that might occur later and when you should call about such symptoms
- Special care for stitches, bandages, or casts
- Whether you should call your pediatrician or a specialist to arrange for follow-up care

Do not hesitate to call the pediatrician if something appears wrong with your child after you go home.

Be a role model

Your child looks to you for clues about how to act. If you are emotionally distraught or squeamish, your child will be more likely to get upset in the emergency room. Do your best to remain calm. If the sight of blood disturbs you, look away. If you feel faint, put your head between your knees or leave the room.

My daughter broke her right wrist, and it caused what they call significant deformation. It was really gross. But while the doctor worked on it, I tried to not register alarm or shock. I kept real impassive features so if she were trying to read my face, I would be more or less inscrutable. When it's my child and I don't want to scare her, I click into warrior mom.

Many parents can hold their emotions in check until their child is out of danger. But don't be surprised if you feel the need to cry when it's all over.

Staying in the hospital

Sometimes a child is too ill or injured to go home after an emergency room visit. Doctors then will recommend that your child be admitted to the hospital. Your child will be moved to another floor and placed in a room, sometimes alone, sometimes with other children. If you wish, you can ask if a private room is available. You might check with your insurance company to find out whether a private room will be covered if it's not considered to be medically necessary.

Again, try to remain with your child if she is admitted. Use the telephone in the room or your cell phone to notify your family, friends, and workplace. If you left the house without clothes, toys, games, or books for your child, ask a family member or friend to collect these items and bring them to the hospital. Also, have them bring a change of clothes and toothbrush for you.

When your child settles in, a nurse will probably come into the room, introduce herself, and take vital signs (blood pressure, heart rate, breathing rate). The nurse may ask you to repeat information that you already gave to the emergency room staff. This may seem repetitive, but you may have forgotten an important detail in the emergency room. It's important for you to provide complete information and answer questions.

The nurse should explain what will happen that night. For example, if your child has a concussion, the nurse may need to wake her up every hour. If the nurse doesn't explain the first night's plan, do not hesitate to ask.

My 7-year-old daughter had a lengthy, complicated seizure, and was admitted to the hospital through the emergency room. I assured her that I would stay with her and take care of her. I told her it might be stressful in the hospital, but we would make time for fun. I talked about how cool it would be to watch TV in bed all day. We found a computer to play with (a big treat) and had my husband bring in games and coloring books. The fun things really helped her cope.

Chapter 3

Preparing Your Child

"You're braver than you believe,
and stronger than you seem,
and smarter than you think."

— Christopher Robin
to Winnie the Pooh

CHILDREN WHO ARE WELL PREPARED for hospital visits often feel comfortable and sometimes even excited about their upcoming hospitalization. But, children who aren't expecting the strange surroundings or discomfort of medical procedures might feel frightened or disoriented. Taking some time to prepare yourself and your child is well worth the effort. More information about preparing your child is in Chapter 8, *Surgery*.

Help from the staff

You can find many resources in the pediatrician's office, at the library, or at the hospital to help prepare your child for his hospital visit. Some doctors provide age-appropriate videos that explain surgery and other procedures in terms children understand.

Many children's hospitals employ child life specialists who can help your child learn about a procedure using dolls or toys. Hospitals also have child psychologists and social workers skilled at explaining how hospitals work and answering children's questions. As soon as you know your child will be spending time in the hospital, ask the doctor about these specialized services.

Matthew was in sixth grade and he was worried about the surgery for putting the catheter in his chest. The child life worker showed him what a catheter looked like, then they explored the pre-op area, the actual surgery room, and post-op. She showed him on a cloth doll exactly where the incision would be and how

13

the scar would look. Then she introduced him to "Fred," the
IV pump. She said that Fred would be going places with him,
and that Fred would keep him from getting so many pokes. She
really helped him with his fears.

Take a tour

A tour can be an excellent way to familiarize your child with the hospital before admission. The tour might include a look at the operating room, an explanation of anesthesia, and an opportunity to talk with children who have undergone similar procedures.

> *Ian was cross-eyed. We had a couple of friends who had eye*
> *procedures done. They both talked to him and told him how*
> *much better they were after surgery. They really set up a feeling*
> *of "I've been through this. It was fine. It was an okay experi-*
> *ence." It helped him a lot.*

If you take a tour, make sure your child also gets to see the fun parts of the hospital, such as the play area and cafeteria. Although adults often cringe at hospital cafeteria food, many children enjoy walking through the line and choosing their own food. It also helps to tell your child some of the positive things about going to the hospital, for example:

- He will not have to do chores.
- She will get her own telephone, television, and remote control.
- He will get to pick his own food off a menu and eat in bed or in a cafeteria.
- She will have buttons to push that make the bed go up and down.

If your child is young, show her that all beds in the hospital—even adults' beds—have rails on the sides.

> *Eighteen-month-old Gylany had the croup. Our pediatrician*
> *sent her to the hospital to spend the night in a humidified tent. I*
> *told her, "We're going to have an adventure today. We are going*
> *to the hospital to get some help for your breathing. We're going*
> *to camp out in a tent there. It will be just like the rain forest,*

but instead of raining on the outside of the tent it will rain on
the inside. I'll stay with you and we'll cuddle in our tent, and
look for rain forest birds and animals." I climbed right into the
tent and we spent the night in our private rain forest.

You might also make the tour part of an educational experience. If your child will return to school shortly after the hospitalization, you or your child can talk to her teacher about letting him do a report or research project on some aspect of hospital life. Asking questions and becoming something of a hospital expert may help your child feel more informed and in control of the situation.

Read books together

Many children enjoy reading age-appropriate books with their parents about going to the hospital. Books offer factual information that may clear up any misconceptions or fears your child has about what happens at the hospital. Reading together also allows time for your child to ask you questions and perhaps share some worries.

You can find helpful books at your local bookstore or in a hospital library. Bookstores often have a children's book expert who knows what's available for each age group. The hospital librarian, social worker, counselor, or child life specialist may also have recommendations. Many suggestions are listed in the *Resources* section at the end of this book.

Before my 4-year-old son went to the hospital, we bought a
book written by Mr. Rogers, called Going to the Hospital.
It showed children and their families in the hospital, during
admission, having x-rays, in bed. It was very reassuring and
informative. Reading books allowed his fears and concerns
to surface. He asked questions he might not have asked if we
hadn't cuddled up on the couch and read the book together.

Older children and teens might look online for information about their illness, treatment, or upcoming procedures. Information online can range from helpful to wildly inaccurate. Mention this to your child and let him know that if he finds something concerning in his research that it's worth discussing with his doctor.

Answer questions

Whether you use books, videos, tours, computer programs, or other methods to prepare your child, it helps to talk and answer any questions that arise. Young children sometimes believe they are going to the hospital as punishment. Explain that this is not the case. You can tell your child that hospitals are special places that help people who are hurt or sick.

Children also may form incorrect impressions or have scary fantasies about what can occur. They can conjure up genuine horrors, and you should try to replace those fearful imaginings with the truth.

> Our children perceive things differently than we do. We've found it's really important to ask them to explain to us what they think is coming. A lot of times we can dispel their fears. Before heart surgeries, we have asked David what he thinks is going to happen. Once he asked, "How do I know they're not going to take my heart out?"

Be realistic. If you tell your child that a painful procedure won't hurt, he won't believe you the next time. Be truthful, and explain the procedure as well as you can. Encourage your child to ask the doctor questions, too.

If your baby must be hospitalized, she can't ask questions or understand explanations. An infant's whole world is eating, sleeping, being held, being sung to, and being nestled in her parent's arms. These familiar comforts will help soothe your baby during medical procedures.

Help with longer-term hospitalization

If your child will be in the hospital or undergoing medical treatments for a long time, a child life specialist can do a great deal to help your child understand and deal with the hospital and medical treatment. Child life specialists provide play experiences that encourage expression of feelings and increase understanding. They also talk with other members of the healthcare team about the emotional needs of children and their families.

Giving children some control over what happens helps tremendously. Many children have definite opinions about how they want things done in the hospital. Encourage your child to express those opinions and do what you can to accommodate them. For example, your child might prefer that you hold her during a procedure, instead of a nurse. Or your child might like a handshake from every doctor who comes in the room. Your child might have a preference for which arm to use for the IV. Chapter 7, *Common Procedures*, has many suggestions for giving your child some control over what happens in the hospital. Children do better when they have choices and when they are prepared.

> *My son and I learned lots from other patients and parents about how to survive a hospital stay. We learned it was okay to wear shorts and T-shirts instead of hospital gowns. We learned parents can sleep on the floor if no cot is available. We learned to welcome all visitors, especially those bringing food. We learned to share our treats with hospital personnel—from the doctors to the cleaning staff. We learned that we could request a favorite nurse. We met friends and had incredible experiences that we will remember all our lives.*

Chapter 4
The Facilities

"Remember that worry will cause much pain
over things that will never happen."

— Thomas Jefferson

WHETHER YOU AND YOUR CHILD are in the hospital for a day or for much longer, the experience can be trying. Hospitals are noisy bureaucracies that run on a time schedule all their own. For a child, being hospitalized means being separated from parents, brothers, sisters, friends, pets, and the comfort and familiarity of home. However, with a little ingenuity, you can make the most of the facilities, liven up the atmosphere, and even have some fun.

Staying with your child

One of the biggest worries a child often has in the hospital is being separated from her parents. If you stay at your child's side, you can provide comfort, entertainment, and advocacy. Whether your child is admitted to a children's hospital or the pediatric floor of a community hospital, the staff usually know how much better most children do when a parent sleeps in the room. The room might have a small couch that converts into a bed, or you can sleep on a cot provided by the hospital.

Sometimes it isn't possible to stay with your child if you are a single parent or if both parents work full time. Many families have grandparents, aunts, uncles, or close friends stay at the hospital when parents cannot be there. Older children and teenagers may not want a parent in the room at night, but they will likely need an advocate there during the day just as much as younger children do.

My daughter has had several major surgeries since she was 15. Generally, the nurses tell me that I cannot stay with her in the room overnight because she is old enough to take care of herself.

Well, I'm a nurse, and in our family, whether you are an adult or child, someone stays with you in the hospital around the clock. So, I just nicely tell them, "I will be quiet, I won't get in your way. As a matter of fact, I'll help out quite a bit. But I am going to stay." And I do.

If your child does not have a cell phone, show her how to use the telephone in the room for times when a family member cannot be present. If he does have a cell phone, make sure it's fully charged. Tape a phone number nearby where you can be reached and instruct your child to call if anyone proposes an unexpected change in treatment. Tell hospital staff that only you can authorize such changes, unless the situation is life-threatening.

Illness and hospitals can make children feel like their bodies are being invaded. Your child may feel better if you take responsibility for some nursing care. Children sometimes prefer parents to help them to the bathroom or to change dirty sheets. If you can make the bed, keep the room tidy, and give back rubs, you will free nurses to spend more time providing medical care for your child.

If you encourage your child to make choices whenever possible, you may help her regain a sense of personal power.

- Older children should be included in all discussions about their treatment.
- Younger children can decide when to take a bath, which arm to use for an IV, what to order for meals, what clothes to wear, and how to decorate the room.
- Some children request a hug or a handshake after all treatments or procedures.

My 4-year-old daughter had to take a lot of medicine when she was in the hospital. But, we let her choose the order she took them in ("white pill first or yellow?") and what to chase it down with (soda was a big treat so it made the pills go down easily!). She picked what she got to wear, what stuffed animal was duct taped to the IV pole, whether she was going to watch TV or listen to music, and when we went for our walks around the hospital. Feeling "in charge" made her feel better.

The room

Hospital rooms are sometimes painted drab colors, and most rooms don't have particularly scenic views. You (and your child if he is well enough) can do a lot to liven up a dull hospital room. If your child's hospital visit will be brief, a few touches of home (e.g., a bright pillowcase, a favorite stuffed animal or toy) probably will suffice. If the visit will be longer, making the room more familiar helps everyone. You can:

• Cover the walls with big, bright posters.

• Tape cards on the walls, hang them from strings like a mobile, or arrange them on the windowsills.

• Put up pictures of the child engaged in her favorite activities. Add photos of family members, friends, and pets.

• Place a favorite stuffed animal, blanket, or quilt on the bed. This can provide great comfort, especially for younger children. But make sure your linens or animals are not accidentally carted away with the soiled linens.

• Make the room smell good with potpourri or aromatherapy oils that your child likes.

• Bring a guest book for each visitor and member of the medical staff to sign. Or put up a sign-in poster for doctors and nurses, who must sign in before they begin examinations or take vital signs. Some children ask staff members to outline their hands on a poster and write inside the hand print.

• Bring music (e.g., on an iPod®, phone, or portable stereo) to block out hospital noise and help everyone relax.

• If there isn't an in-room DVD player, check to see if you can sign one out from the hospital's media library, or bring a laptop. You can watch a favorite funny movie or TV show because belly laughs help.

• Bring clothes from home. Most hospitals provide brightly colored smocks for young patients, but many children and teens prefer to wear their own clothing. This can pose a laundry problem, so check to see if the floor has washers available for families.

- Bring in age-appropriate games, puzzles, books, and things that make kids laugh (e.g., joke books or Silly String®).

> *The first thing we did was put up a poster of the Little Engine that Could saying, "I think I can. I think I can." Then we covered every square inch of the walls of 3-year-old Meagan's room with colorful posters. We tried to use ones with depth so it would seem like the room was larger. We hung up all of her cards from her preschool friends. Balloons covered the ceiling. The room was colorful and full.*

Taking a tour of the floor as soon as you get there really helps. During the tour, you'll be able to find out if a microwave and refrigerator are available, what the sleeping arrangements for parents are, and where you shower. Try to get a hospital handbook if one is available. These booklets often include information on billing, parking, discounts, and other helpful tips.

Playing

Children need to play, especially when hospitalized. The hospital might have a recreation therapy or child life department that has toys, books, dolls, and crafts, and is staffed by specialists who really know how to play with children. These staff members may also provide therapeutic activities, such as medical play with dolls, which helps children express fears or concerns about what is happening to them.

> *When I wanted to have a conference with the doctor about Katy's treatment, I called recreation therapy and they sent two wonderful ladies to the room. The doctor and I were able to talk privately, and Katy had a great time making herself a gold crown and decorating her wheelchair with streamers and jewels.*

The fun-filled activities and smiling staff people in the recreation therapy rooms are a cheerful change from lying in a hospital bed. If your child needs to stay in bed or is too ill to go to the play area, you can arrange for a child life specialist to bring a bundle of toys, games, and books to the room. Music therapists might also come by the room to visit. This can give you time to go out to eat or take a walk.

Sometimes you can create your own fun with just a little imagination. On one particular occasion, Matthew was feeling especially bored. With a little ingenuity, we soon discovered that four unused IV poles and as many blankets as we could "steal" from the linen cart made for one pretty cool tent. We then used the mattress from a roll-away cot, and spent the night "camping" in his hospital room. He had a wonderful time.

Exercise is important, too. For kids strong enough to walk, exploring the hospital can be fun. Even if your child can't walk, you can wheel her around in a wheelchair, pull her in a wagon, or push the IV pole down the hall with her standing on the base of it. (This is also a great workout for you.) You can also:

- Plan a daily excursion to the gift shop or the cafeteria

- Go outside and walk the perimeter of the hospital if weather and the neighborhood permit

- Climb the stairs to the roof to feel the sun on your face

Tori was sick and could not go trick or treating one year. When she was in the hospital after Halloween, we went reverse trick or treating. I brought in her witch costume and she ran around the hospital giving out candy to her therapists, nurses, and doctors. It was fabulous. She looked so cute. People in the halls did think it was a little weird but staff members understood that you do what makes you happy. Just call November 16th Halloween and everyone just pretends it is.

Food

The hospital will provide meals for your child. But you must eat as well and buying meals day after day in the hospital cafeteria can get expensive.

- Check to see if the floor has a refrigerator, microwave, or kitchen for patient use. Because children often want to eat between meals, such facilities are handy to heat hot chocolate, make popcorn, or cook leftovers.

- Put your name in a prominent place on your containers.
- Ask family members and friends to bring food when they visit.
- Find out which local restaurants deliver take-out food to hospital rooms.
- Consider ordering extra items to come up on your child's tray.

> Our hospital provides vouchers for the cafeteria that can be used instead of ordering food for the room. For us, they have been a godsend. The food on the tray is much worse than what is in the cafeteria. When our son is not able to go to the cafeteria, we go down and bring the food back to his room.

Parking

Emergency rooms usually have special parking spots in front of the entrance, but finding regular parking near hospitals is sometimes difficult. The hospital might have both long-term and short-term parking arrangements. The nurses and other parents will know whether parking passes are available or where the cheapest parking is located.

> I had no idea that the hospital gave out free parking passes to their frequent customers. Now I tell every new parent to check as soon as possible to see if they can get a parking pass. It will save them lots of money that they would have spent on meters and parking tickets, and time that they would have spent running out to move the car out of the emergency parking spot.

Waiting

You can expect lengthy waits for everything from routine tests to surgery. Many parents find themselves getting nervous or angry in large teaching hospitals while waiting for the doctors to appear during rounds each morning (i.e., when attending physicians, residents, and interns move from room to room in a large group), then feel let down when the visit lasts only a few moments. If you have questions, write them down and tell the doctors when they come in that you would like a few moments to talk with them.

Some young children become upset when large groups of doctors or nurses come in during rounds. If this bothers your child, request that only your doctor and assigned nurse be admitted. You have the right to refuse to have student doctors in the room if you feel that their presence is not helpful for your child.

Even if your child is in a community hospital, you may have to wait for your doctor or the doctor employed by the hospital (called a "hospitalist"). If you become frustrated, call your doctor's office to get an estimate of when he will arrive or ask a nurse when the hospitalist is most likely to come by.

> It seemed like we spent most of the years of treatment waiting to see a doctor who was running hours behind schedule, so I came well prepared. I always carried a large bag containing an assortment of things to eat and drink, toys to play with, coloring books and markers, books to read, and Play-Doh®. My son stayed occupied and we avoided many problems. I saw too many parents expecting their bored children to sit still and be quiet for long periods of time.

The hospital might have TVs, DVDs, and games available in recreational therapy rooms, or you may need to bring your own things. Have your child pick out favorite card games, board games, computer games, drawing materials, and books.

> You don't have to go too crazy. Make sure you watch the videos or eat the popcorn or flirt with the nurses or taunt the residents or leave notes for the cleaning lady or chat with the security guard or make coffee for all the parents or pretend you like puking or show the nurses how to hack into the hospital mainframe or paint your face with Butt Paste. Or, all of the above, if you like. Just do something.

Chapter 5

The Staff

*"Diagnosis is not the end,
but the beginning of practice."*
— Martin H. Fischer

IN LARGE HOSPITALS, a steady parade of people—doctors, nurses, medical students, nursing students, lab technicians, child psychologists, child life specialists, and more—come in and out of the room. Understanding the hospital hierarchy can help you sort out who is responsible for your child's care.

The doctors

As with people in any other profession, doctors have many different specialties, temperaments, and skill levels. Your child's treatment will be greatly enhanced if you and your child trust and communicate well with the doctor. The majority of discussions and decision-making will take place with the primary care doctor and your child's specialist.

- **Primary care doctor.** Your child's primary care doctor (usually a pediatrician or family practice doctor) oversees all medical care. When your child is in the hospital, the primary care physician typically will visit, get reports from specialists, and check on your child. She should also be available to answer questions and provide support.

- **Specialist.** A specialist has extensive training in a specific area of medicine. Cardiologists, for example, specialize in hearts; orthopedists specialize in bones and joints.

Your child may see many other doctors if she is in a teaching hospital. To help you sort them out, here's a list of who's who in large, children's hospitals:

- **Medical student.** A medical student is a college graduate who is attending medical school. Medical students wear white coats, but do not have M.D. on their name tags.

- **Intern.** An intern (sometimes called a first-year resident) is a graduate of medical school who is in his or her first year of postgraduate training.

- **Resident.** A resident is a graduate of medical school in her second to sixth year of postgraduate training. Most residents at pediatric hospitals will be pediatricians upon completion of their residencies.

- **Fellow.** A fellow is a doctor who has completed four years of medical school, several years of residency, and is taking additional specialty training.

- **Attending physician.** An attending physician (called simply "attending") is above a fellow in the hospital hierarchy. Medical centers hire these well-established specialists to provide and oversee medical care and to train interns, residents, and fellows. They are frequently also professors on the staff of an affiliated medical school.

Residents usually rotate to different floors every four weeks, so they are an ever-changing group. The fellow or attending assigned to your child will be most familiar with your child's situation and is the best person to seek out if questions arise about your child's treatment or illness.

If your child is at a community hospital, her primary care doctor or a doctor who only works in the hospital (called "hospitalist") will provide most of her care. But if your child is at a teaching hospital, she will be assigned a doctor from the appropriate specialty. These physicians will care for your child throughout treatment.

The nurses

Nurses are an essential part of the hospital hierarchy. Several nurses with different levels of training may all play a role in your child's treatment.

- **Nurse assistant or aide.** A nurse assistant can take vital signs (heart rate, breathing rate, blood pressure), perform hygiene care, or change bedding.

- **Licensed practical nurse (LPN).** LPNs take vital signs, give medications, and perform general care under the supervision of a registered nurse.

- **Registered nurse (RN).** An RN has a bachelor's or associate's degree in nursing, then takes a licensing examination. These medical professionals give medicines, take vital signs, start and monitor IVs, and communicate changes in condition to doctors.

- **Nurse practitioner or clinical nurse specialist.** A nurse practitioner is a registered nurse who has completed an educational program that covers advanced skills. In some hospitals and clinics, nurse practitioners perform procedures, such as spinal taps.

- **Head nurse or charge nurse.** A head nurse supervises all the nurses on the floor for one shift.

- **Clinical nurse manager.** A clinical nurse manager is the administrator for an entire floor, unit, or clinic.

> At our hospital, each of our nurses is different, but each is wonderful. They simply love the kids. They listen to the kids, throw parties, and act as counselor, best friend, stern parent. They hug moms and dads. They cry. I have come to respect them so much because they have such a hard job to do, and they do it so well.

Other staff members

Many other staff members will help you and your child during your stay in the hospital.

- **Interpreter.** You have a legal right to an interpreter if you have limited ability to speak or understand English. You have the right to understand what is being said about what is happening with your child's health. The healthcare workers need to know what you and your child are saying so they can provide the best care.

- **Psychologist.** Child psychologists help children and families cope with and adjust to illness, injury, and hospitalization. They frequently supervise members of the other helping professionals such as social workers and child life professionals.

- **Child life specialist.** These professionals help children cope through play, preparation, education, and self-expression activities. They also provide emotional support for all family members by providing information, support, and guidance.

- **Social worker.** These professionals educate children and parents about all aspects of hospitalization, facilitate communication with other members of the healthcare team, provide crisis intervention if needed, and refer families to hospital and community resources.

- **Chaplain.** Most hospitals have chaplains on staff who are available for counseling, religious services, prayer, and other types of spiritual support.

- **Discharge planner.** The hospital discharge planner will meet with you to discuss when your child will be discharged, whether any services are needed at home (e.g., physical therapy), and if referral to an appropriate home care agency or support organization is needed.

Working with the staff

Many wonderful and some not-so-wonderful people work in hospitals. Parents sometimes find that their anxiety makes them less tolerant of inefficiency or confusion. Your child will feel more secure if you work with hospital staff rather than becoming adversarial. If you help change your child's soiled bedding, take out food trays, and give baths, you will free overworked nurses to take care of medicines and IVs. Nurses are usually happy to answer questions or explain planned treatments or procedures to you and your child.

Some parents recommend introducing themselves and their child to the nurse and residents on each shift. You might add that you'll help as much as you can. If they are not too busy, talk with them about matters unrelated to the hospital. Establishing a personal relationship makes everyone feel more comfortable and connected. Try to thank them for any kind words or deeds.

> *Give staff a chance to see your child as a human being. Show pictures. "This is the little kid who likes Barney. He loves to play this song. This is what he looks like when he's not all puffed up from steroids." They see so many kids who are so sick every day. It's important for them to see that sparkle in your child's eye.*

Shift changes

As soon as you can, learn about the shift changes on your child's floor. These generally occur every eight or twelve hours. Shift change is a necessary, and sometimes hectic, time when the outgoing staff members meet with the incoming staff to report on the status of all the patients on the floor. They discuss:

- A brief history of each patient

- A summary of major events from the last two shifts, such as, "She vomited after each dose of morphine, so today we switched to Tylenol® with codeine and she's feeling much better."

- What needs to be done, for example, "The lab work is not done yet and Dr. Jones is waiting for the results."

- Family information, such as, "John's father had to go to work. His phone number is posted by the bed. John's aunt is staying with him now."

After hearing a report on all the patients, the nurses decide how to assign patients to incoming nurses to keep the work load even. Next, each nurse spends a few minutes organizing and prioritizing what he needs to do for each of his patients.

You should try to avoid calling during the shift change hour (a half hour before and a half hour after) with non-urgent questions, comments, or requests. If you press the call button, the unit secretary will tell you it may be a while before a nurse comes because, "They are in report." Of course, the nurses will respond to things that cannot wait, such as your child vomiting, an empty IV bag, severe pain, or another emergency.

Whenever Katy is hospitalized, I introduce myself and my daughter and ask when the shift change is. Then I say, "I'll do my best not to bother you." I always get a grateful smile. If I need something and I see them in report, I wave and go back into the room. I get more smiles. Then, whenever I really need help, they are almost always just fabulous. I've found that when we all work as a team, it goes much smoother.

Chapter 6

Communicating
with Doctors

*"There is only one rule for being a good
talker—learn to listen."*

— Christopher Morley

COMMUNICATING WELL WITH YOUR DOCTOR can mean the difference between a very good relationship and a very poor one. Good communication can improve your child's care and put your mind at ease. Poor communication can leave doctors, parents, and children feeling frustrated or resentful.

Types of relationships

Three types of relationships tend to develop between doctors and parents:

- **Paternal.** In a paternal relationship, the parent is submissive, and the doctor assumes a parental role. This dynamic may seem desirable to parents who are uncomfortable or inexperienced in dealing with medical issues, but it places all the responsibility for decisions on the doctor. Doctors are human. If your child's doctor makes a mistake and you are not monitoring drugs and treatments, these mistakes may go unnoticed. You are the expert on your child and you know best how to gauge his reactions to drugs and treatments.

  I once asked a fellow about the results of my daughter's blood work. She literally patted me on the head and said it was her job to worry about that, not mine. I said in a nice voice that I thought it was a reasonable question and that I would appreciate an answer.

Some parents are intimidated by doctors and fear that if they question the doctors their child will suffer. This type of behavior robs the child of an adult advocate who speaks up when something seems wrong.

- **Adversarial.** Some parents adopt an "us against them" attitude, which is counterproductive. They seem to feel the illness and any discomforts of treatment are the fault of the medical staff, and they blame staff for any setbacks that occur. This attitude undermines the child's confidence in her doctors and nurses, which is a crucial part of healing.

- **Collegial.** This is a true partnership in which parents and doctors respect each other. The doctor recognizes that the parents are the experts on their own child. The parents respect the doctor's knowledge and feel comfortable discussing treatment options or concerns that arise.

Honest communication is necessary for this partnership to work, but the effort is well worth it. The child has confidence in her doctor, the parents have lessened their stress by creating a supportive relationship with the doctor, and the doctor feels comfortable that the family will comply with the treatment plan.

> *Early in my daughter's illness, we changed pediatricians. The first was aloof and patronizing, and the second was smart, warm, funny, and caring. He was a constant bright spot in our lives through some dark times. So every year, my two daughters put on their Santa hats and bring homemade cookies to the pediatrician and nurse. The first year, she was so weak I had to carry her in. She and her sister looked them in the eye and sang, "We Wish You a Merry Christmas." Her nurse went in the back room and cried, and her doctor got misty-eyed. I'll always be thankful for their care.*

Communication

Clear and frequent communication is the foundation of a positive doctor/parent relationship. Doctors need to be able to explain clearly and listen well, and parents need to feel comfortable asking questions and expressing concerns before they grow into grievances. Nurses and doctors cannot read parents' minds, nor can parents prepare their child for a procedure unless it has been explained well. The following are parent suggestions about how to establish and maintain good communication with your child's healthcare team.

- Tell the staff how much you want to know.

  I told them the first day to treat me like a medical student. I asked them to share all information, current studies, lab results, everything, with me. I told them, in advance, that I hoped they wouldn't be offended by lots of questions, because knowledge was comfort to me.

- Inform staff of your child's temperament, likes, and dislikes.

- Encourage a close relationship between your child and his doctor, and don't let anyone talk in front of your child as if she is not there. Marina Rozen observes in *Advice to Doctors and Other Big People:*

  "The best part about the doctor is when he gives me bubble gum. The worst part is when he's in the room with me and my mom and he only talks to my mom. I've told him I don't like that, but he doesn't listen."

- Try to form a warm relationship with your child's nurse. Most children's hospitals assign each patient a primary nurse who will oversee all care. Nurses usually possess vast knowledge and experience about both medical and practical aspects of treatment. Often, nurses can resolve misunderstandings between doctor and parents.

  We found that sitting down and talking things over with the nurses helped immensely. They were very familiar with each drug and its side effects. They told us many stories about children who had been through the same thing and were doing well years later. They always seemed to have time to give encouragement, a smile, or a hug.

- Ask for definitions of unfamiliar terms. Repeat back the information to ensure that you understood correctly. Don't hesitate to write down answers or tape-record conferences. If taping, it is helpful to say, "I hope you don't mind, but I have trouble remembering all of the information. This will help me keep everything straight." That way, the doctors are not put on the defensive and you'll have what you need.

- Keep a written list of questions by the bedside. This practice will help you remember what to ask and prevent lots of follow-up conversations.

- Make sure that every person who comes in the room thoroughly washes his or her hands. Hospitals are germy places and doctors, nurses, physical therapists, and many others go from room to room all day. So, politely stop anyone from touching your child or your child's belongings (no hugging that teddy bear) until hand washing is complete.

- Make sure you know what medication or treatment is scheduled for each day. Make the final checks on all drugs whenever possible (check that it is the right drug, the correct dosage, and that your child's name is on the syringe or bag).

> When my daughter was in the hospital one time, the nurse came in with two syringes. I asked what they were, and she said immunizations. I said that it must be a mistake, and the nurse said that the orders were in the chart. So I checked my daughter's chart, and the orders were there, but they had another child's name on them.

- Seek the best staff person to perform a procedure. The medical team includes many specialists: doctors, nurses, physical therapists, x-ray technicians, and more. At training hospitals, many of these people will be in the early stages of their careers. If a procedure is not going well, you can tell the person to stop and ask for a more skilled person to do the job.

- Know your rights, and the hospital's. Legally, your child cannot be treated without your permission. If a doctor suggests a procedure that you do not feel comfortable with, keep asking questions until you feel fully informed. You have the right to refuse the procedure if you do not think it is necessary.

> One day in the hospital, a group of fellows came in and announced that they were going to do a lung biopsy on Jesse. I told them that I hadn't heard anything about it from her

attending, and I just didn't think it was the right thing to do. They said, "We have to do it," and I repeated that I just didn't think it needed to be done until we talked to the attending. They seemed angry, but we stood our ground. When the attending came later, he said that they were not supposed to do a biopsy because the surgeon said it was too risky of an area in the lung to get to.

If the hospital staff feels that you are wrongfully withholding permission for treatment, they can take you to court. All parties should remember that the most important person is the child.

Creating positive relationships

A positive relationship between parents and doctors depends on clear and frequent communication. Doctors should explain clearly and listen well, and parents should feel comfortable asking questions and expressing concerns before they become grievances. Here are a few suggestions from parents:

• Treat doctors with respect, and expect respect from them.

• Recognize that you are under stress and so are doctors and nurses. Do not blame them for your child's illness or explode in anger. Be an advocate, not an adversary.

• Request a conference if you have something to discuss with the doctor that will take time. These are routinely scheduled between parents and physicians, and should allow enough time for a thorough discussion. Grabbing a busy doctor in the hallway is unfair to him, and may result in an unsatisfactory answer to you.

• Negotiate. You have a right to a conversation with the doctor about your wishes. Tell her what you would like to see happen, and discuss all of the options. You may be able to work out a mutually acceptable plan.

• Try to be genuinely friendly and helpful. Then, if a problem arises or you need help, your good relationship with staff will help you get a positive response.

• Show appreciation. A short thank-you note or a plate of cookies to a doctor or nurse will be warmly received.

I sent thank-you notes to three residents after my daughter's first hospitalization. The notes were short but sweet. I wanted them to know how much we appreciated their many kindnesses.

• • • • •

I always try to thank the nurse or doctor when they apologize for being late and give the reason. I don't mind waiting if it is for a good cause, and I feel they show respect when they apologize.

Conflict resolution

Conflict is a part of life. In a situation where a child's health is threatened, the heightened emotions and frequent involvement with medical bureaucracy mean that conflicts can easily arise. Because conflicts are common, resolving them is crucial. A speedy resolution might result if you adopt Henry Ford's motto, "Don't find fault, find a remedy."

• Recognize that speaking up is difficult, especially if being assertive is uncomfortable for you.

> *I wanted to stay with Meara when she had her stitches, but the doctor was concerned that I was going to faint. So I said, "Is there anything I can do to make you more comfortable about me staying with her?" He asked, "Can you sit in a chair?" I said, "Of course." He heard what I needed, and we negotiated an agreeable solution. I sat on a chair holding my daughter's hand, and he stitched her up without worrying that I was going to fall flat on the ground.*

• Be specific and nonconfrontational when describing problems. For example, "My son gets very nervous the longer we wait for the doctor. The doctor came by the room three hours after he said he would. Could we ask someone next time to see if the doctor is on schedule? Who should we ask?" rather than, "Do you think your time is more valuable than mine?"

• Use "I" statements. For example, "I feel upset when you won't answer my questions," rather than, "You never listen to me."

- Assume mistakes will happen—only vigilance will prevent them. Try to be tactful when you point out errors.

- Ask a hospital social worker or psychologist for advice on problem solving. Their job includes serving as mediators between staff and parents. If the issue is not resolved, you can contact the hospital's ethics consultant.

- Teach your child to speak her mind. If you need to leave the room briefly, make sure you have coached your child on what to expect while you are gone.

> My two children, Sean and Angie, have had many hospi-
> talizations for minor injuries (stitches and casts) and major
> procedures (benign tumor removed from chest, abdominal
> surgery). I have taught them to be pleasant but firm in their
> dealings with staff. They are good at saying, "Excuse me, but
> we need to wait until my mom gets here," or "No, I don't want
> that done now." I have taught them that they are in charge of
> their own bodies. I'm proud to say that although they are never
> mean or threatening, they have learned to express themselves
> with clarity and firmness.

Chapter 7

Common Procedures

"Mommy, I didn't cry but my eyes got bright."
— A 4-year-old after
a procedure

IF YOUR CHILD IS IN THE HOSPITAL for an emergency or for a very short stay, some procedures are inevitable—from blood draws to injections of medications. One or both parents should try to be present during all procedures, especially for small children. Parents set the tone. A calm parent and a well-prepared child create the best likelihood for a quick, peaceful procedure.

Preparation

You can discuss when and how to prepare your child for upcoming procedures with the child life specialist or nurse. Consider how much advance notice to give your child before procedures. You may want to experiment. Some children do better with several days to prepare, while others just spend the time worrying. Many child life specialists accompany children to procedures and stay to provide support. Sometimes, a child's needs change if treatment lasts a long time, so good communication and flexibility are essential.

> For Christie, playing "procedures" helped release many feelings. We stocked a medical kit with gauze pads, tape, tubing, stethoscope, reflex hammer, and pretend needles and syringes. We made IV bottles from empty shampoo containers, complete with tubing and plastic needles. Many dolls and stuffed animals in our house fell apart after being subject to many shots, IVs, and surgeries.

If you find that you are unable to help your child during procedures, ask the child life specialist or other member of the healthcare team to be present to comfort your child.

Taking pills

If your child needs to swallow pills or liquid medications, it will probably be much easier if you try to get off to a good start and establish cooperation early. You can experiment with different techniques to find what works best for her.

• Taste each medication. If it tastes all right, tell your child. Many pills can be chewed or swallowed whole without taste problems.

• If a liquid medication tastes bad, you can ask the pharmacist about FLAVORx® flavorings that are mixed with the medication (for information about FLAVORx®, call 1-800-884-5771 or visit *www.flavorx.com*). FLAVORx® come in many flavors that kids like, such as cherry, bubblegum, or orange.

• Ask a nurse or doctor for gel caps and pack pills inside (break them up if necessary). Gel caps come in many sizes, and #4s are small enough for a three- or four-year-old to swallow. They are useful for any medication that bothers your child.

> *I wanted Katy (3 years old) to feel like we were a team right from the first night. So I made a big deal out of tasting each of her medications and pronouncing it good. Thank goodness I tasted the prednisone first. It was nauseating—bitter, metallic, with a lingering aftertaste. I asked the nurse for some small gel caps, and packed them with the pills which I had broken in half. I gave Katy her choice of drinks to take her pills with and taught her to swallow gel caps with a large sip of liquid.*

• Give your child a choice of drinks to help swallow a pill or gel cap. Ask the doctor or pharmacist first, though, because some pills should not be taken with certain liquids (e.g., milk, grapefruit juice).

• Suggest that your child hold his nose while he swallows medication that has a bad taste or smell.

• Allow your child to mix pills with other food, such as chocolate chips.

• Crush pills in a small amount of pudding, applesauce, jam, frozen juice concentrate, or other favorite food. This is especially effective with smaller children. Ask the doctor or pharmacist first, though, because some pills should not be crushed (e.g., time-release pills).

Jeremy was 4 when he was hospitalized, and we used to crush up the pills and mix them with ice cream. This worked well for us.

• Let your child experiment with ways to take liquid medication, such as sipping from a dosing cup or squirting from a syringe into the mouth followed by a drink of a favorite beverage (e.g., juice).

• Give your child choices, such as, "Do you want the pink pill or the six white pills first?"

Children usually associate taking medicine with being sick, so you may have to explain if they must continue taking pills even if they feel well. Some parents say to young children, "The pills are needed to gobble up the last few germs." Others explain that medicine can prevent the illness from returning.

Teenagers face different issues with taking pills than do small children. Although many teenagers are responsible about taking their medication, with others problems arise because adolescence is a time of growing independence and separation from parents. A doctor, nurse, or social worker may be able to help the teen understand why it is important to take all prescribed medicines.

Giving children all required medications is very important. Many studies show the dangers of not finishing all medications, such as the illness returning or the evolution of drug-resistant infections.

Taking a temperature

Your child's temperature will likely be taken many times during a hospital stay to check for a fever.

There are several ways to take temperatures: under the tongue, on the side of the forehead, or in the ear using a special type of thermometer. The American Academy of Pediatrics (AAP) advises to always use a digital thermometer, never a mercury thermometer. In fact, the AAP recommends that parents should remove mercury thermometers from their homes because mercury is poisonous.

- Digital thermometers can be purchased at any drug store and used under the tongue or under the arm. Some have an alarm that beeps when it is time to remove the thermometer.

- A temporal artery thermometer reads the infrared heat waves released by the temporal artery, which runs across the forehead just below the skin.

- Tympanic, or ear, thermometers measure infrared waves and are very easy to use. These require proper technique to be accurate, so keep the directions handy.

Before your child leaves the hospital, ask your doctor whether you should monitor for fever. Some fever medicines, including aspirin, can interfere with other drugs or cause complications. Find out from your doctor whether you should give medication for fever and how high the fever can go before you call.

> *After six-year-old Kurt's hydrocele surgery, I had to take his temperature frequently for several days. He absolutely refused to have a thermometer in his mouth. It was just impossible, so we compromised and used a digital thermometer under his arm. He complied because he liked to hear the beep at the end.*

X-rays

Few children grow up without having x-rays to check for a broken bone or to look for cavities in teeth. If your child needs an x-ray, ask the doctor or x-ray technician to explain it thoroughly before you proceed. After the explanation, the technician will position your child on an x-ray table with the machine angled over him to get the best view. For a chest x-ray, your child will be strapped in a seated position.

Positioning an injured limb for x-rays may sometimes be painful. Most technicians try to minimize the pain, but you may have to explain to your child that he may be uncomfortable for a few moments while the technician positions his broken limb. Make sure that your child understands the x-ray itself will not hurt.

The technician will place a heavy lead apron over the rest of the child's body to avoid exposure to radiation.

> *My four-year-old daughter Claire needed sinus x-rays. I asked the technician to shield her chest and thyroid, but they didn't have a shield her size. When the technician there tried to minimize my concerns by comparing x-rays to radiation exposure from a television, I told her that I was a radiation therapist and I knew better. So, we ended up having the technician stay in the room, holding the adult shield in front of Claire's thyroid and chest, while the x-ray was taken.*

When your child is in place, the technician will leave the room and will ask you to do the same. Parents and technicians usually can watch the child through a window and often there is a two-way intercom. Explaining the window and intercom can help your child stay calm.

Some children enjoy looking at their x-rays. If your child shows an interest, ask whether the doctor or technician can display the x-rays and give an explanation—it's a fun chance for your child to look at her insides.

Casts

Casts keep broken bones immobile until they mend. They now are lighter and more manageable than the old-fashioned white plaster casts. The doctor may even give your child a choice of colors for his cast.

If your child needs to use a sling with the cast, you should ask for a demonstration on how to use it. Before you leave, you'll be given any special instructions, including whether the cast needs to be kept dry, how long your child must use crutches, and when to return for a checkup. If your child is old enough, she'll probably appreciate being included in the discussion on taking care of the cast.

When it's time to remove the cast, you can ask how it will be done. Often doctors use a small saw that is noisy and can frighten a young child. Ask the doctor to explain that it won't hurt your child's skin. A demonstration might help your child feel comfortable about having the case removed. It's also a good idea to explain that it might be stinky under the cast and skin might be white and wrinkly, but it will look normal in a few days.

> Eight-year-old Sean broke his arm horribly while playing. The orthopedic surgeon put on a plaster cast from wrist to armpit. It needed to be elevated at night, so we rigged up an apparatus above the couch, and Sean slept there. They put on a lightweight blue cast after the first month, followed by a bright yellow one. His friends wrote all over them. Sean was nervous about the big round saw that they used to remove the casts. I told him that he would feel some pressure, and some tickling, but no pain. We sang songs as they removed each cast.

Stitches

Stitches are becoming less common for some injuries and surgeries as new options become available, including staples, butterfly bandages, and skin adhesive. You might consider whether to bring in a plastic surgeon if your child needs stitches on his face or if he could lose some function, such as from a hand injury. Unless the situation is life-threatening, there is usually time to discuss options.

> Ten-year-old Sean fell and cut his forehead down to the bone. I took him to the emergency room and told them that he scars easily and we needed a plastic surgeon to do the repair. They resisted; I insisted. We ended up waiting four hours. The plastic surgeon sprayed on an anesthetic then waited a few minutes before giving the shots of anesthetic. Sean didn't feel a thing, which was good because the wound required many internal and surface stitches. The scar is now so faint that you don't notice it.

Ask the doctor or nurse to explain to your child how the wound will be closed. If shots of anesthetic will be used, the doctor or nurse should tell your child why and how many of the shots are needed. Time spent on preparation is well worth it.

As with any medical procedure, you should get written instructions for care of stitches. Instructions might include ways to keep the stitches dry and the wound from becoming infected.

Sean was worried about having his stitches removed. So I got
some fabric and thread and put in some stitches. I showed him
with scissors how the doctor could cut the stitch and not hurt
the fabric. He felt fine about it after my demonstration.

Starting an IV

Most children's hospitals have teams of technicians who specialize
in starting IVs and drawing blood. They are usually extremely good
at their jobs. An IV technician will generally use a vein in the lower
arm or hand. First, the technician puts a constricting band above
the site to make the veins larger and easier to see and feel. The technician then finds the vein, cleans the area, and inserts the needle.
Sometimes a needle is left in place and sometimes it is removed, leaving only a thin, plastic tube in the vein. The technician makes sure
the needle (or tube) is in the proper place, then covers the site with a
clear dressing, and secures it with tape. Some ways you can help are:

- **Keep your child calm.** The body reacts to fear by constricting
  the blood vessels near the skin surface. The calmer the child is, the
  larger his veins will be. Small children are usually calmest with a
  parent present; teenagers may or may not desire privacy. Listening
  to music, visualizing a tranquil scene (mountains covered with
  snow, floating in a pool), or using the same technician each time
  helps some children.

- **Keep your child warm.** Cold temperatures cause the surface
  blood vessels to constrict. Wrapping the child in a blanket and
  putting a hot water bottle on the arm can enlarge the veins.

- **Encourage your child to drink lots of fluids.** Hydration
  increases the fluid in the veins and makes them easier to find.

- **Let gravity help.** If your child is lying in bed, have her hang her
  arm over the side to increase the size of the vessels in the arm and
  hand.

- **Give your child choices.** If your child has a preference, let him
  pick the arm for the IV. If your child is a veteran of many IVs, let
  her point out the best vein.

- **Tell your child that it's okay to say ouch, squeeze your hand hard, or cry.** Don't say, "It won't hurt," because it does.

- **Stop if problems develop.** The secret to treating children is to spend lots of time on preparation and very little time on procedures. If a conflict arises between your child and the technician or doctor, side with your child. It's far better to take a time-out and regroup than to force the issue and lose your child's trust. Children can be remarkably cooperative if doctors and parents respect their needs and listen to their wishes.

  David was poked many, many times one night and the technician could not get an IV in. We told him to stop. We said, "This child is totally blue from screaming. He's worn out." In the morning we asked the staff for the person who never misses. They brought her in and she got it on the first try.

- **Use topical anesthetics.** If your child needs long-term treatments that include many IVs or blood draws, ask about EMLA®, an anesthetic cream available by prescription. EMLA® is applied to the skin, covered with an airtight bandage, and left on for an hour to anesthetize the skin and underlying tissue.

The advice for starting an IV also applies to drawing blood from the arm. Blood is usually drawn from the large vein on the inside of the elbow using a procedure similar to starting an IV, except that the needle is removed rather than left in the arm.

  When my friends' four-year-old son was very sick, they asked me to bring him a bag of gift-wrapped things. I went to the dollar store and bought a whole bunch of little gifts and wrapped each one. They were things that he could carry into the exam room. Every time the doctor did a needle poke for blood work, he was allowed to open a gift. He loved the four tiny plastic frogs.

Questions to ask

You may be able to save your child some discomfort by avoiding unnecessary tests or procedures. Plus, the more you understand about what is proposed and why it is necessary, the better you can explain it to your child. When your doctor proposes a test, the following are some questions you might ask before giving your consent.

- What is the purpose of the test?
- Does our insurance cover it?
- Are any risks associated with this test?
- What are the possible side effects and how often do they occur?
- Would you describe exactly what will happen during the test?
- Are there special instructions to follow before or after the test?
- When will the results be available?

Many tests can be done at a lab before your child is admitted to the hospital, and the costs might be significantly lower. Ensure that the results of all tests done before hospitalization are sent to the hospital to prevent the need for repeated testing.

> My seven-year-old daughter needed an EEG [electroencephalogram] test that measures the electrical activity in the brain. I asked the technician many pointed questions: What kind of room would she be in? Would other kids be there? Would she be on a bed or bench? Could I stay with her? How many electrodes would be attached to her head, and how would this be done? Would they need to shave any hair? How long does it last? Are there scary or painful parts? Is the machine loud or quiet? After I shared this information with my daughter and answered her questions, the procedure went well. I ended up getting up on the table and lying down next to her to provide some comfort.

Chapter 8

Surgery

"Next to excellence is the appreciation of it."
— William Makepeace
Thackeray

As with most medical procedures, you can do a great deal to make surgery easier for your child. Preparation and communication are crucial before the surgery, as is planning for what comes after surgery.

Educating yourself

In an emergency, you might not have time to ask questions or to meet the surgeon. But, for nonemergency surgeries, you will usually have time to identify the surgeon and hospital that can best help your child.

You can learn about the proposed surgery from your child's pediatrician and by reading any information she provides. During this discussion, you can also ask which hospital and pediatric surgeon she recommends. Children are often sent to large children's hospitals for surgery because community hospitals sometimes do not have surgeons and staff members who specialize in treating children.

After talking with your pediatrician and reading about the surgery, you will probably have some questions. It helps to make a list of your questions so you do not forget any. When you first meet the surgeon, don't hesitate to ask all of your questions so you understand what is being proposed. Many parents tape record or write down the surgeon's answers so they can review them later. The surgeon may provide a video or pamphlet that describes the surgery or you can get this information from a nurse or child life specialist.

*My son had a cavernous angioma, which is an abnormal col-
lection of blood vessels in the brain. Unfortunately, the location
of the angioma was quite poor, deep in the frontal lobe, so very
near the speech center. This is a rare thing in children, so I did
some investigation. I asked my local neurosurgeon who he recommended for a second opinion, and I did a literature search to
see who had published articles on this condition. There was one
vascular neurosurgeon's name that came up more often than
others, and I contacted him by email. He was very responsive
and kind to me immediately. When we travelled 1,000 miles to
meet with him at a large children's hospital, he told us that he
could perform this surgery without any danger of our son losing
his ability to talk. He told us to be prepared for a week in the
hospital, but my son was up talking immediately, and he was
walking within 6 hours of surgery. He ate a breakfast burrito
8 hours after surgery and we were discharged less than 24
hours after surgery. He had just a small bandage, otherwise you
would not know that he had undergone a major operation.*

Some parents recommend checking to make sure that the surgeon
and anesthesiologist are board certified. This means that the doctor
has passed rigorous written and oral tests given by a board of
examiners in his or her specialty. You can call the American Board of
Medical Specialties at (866) ASK-ABMS (275-2267) or visit *https://
www.certificationmatters.org/is-your-doctor-board-certified/search-now.
aspx* to find out if your child's surgeon and anesthesiologist are board
certified.

*We had a bad experience with an anesthesiologist and decided
that from then on, we would choose our own, rather than be
assigned one. I wanted someone competent and compassionate,
who would talk to my teenage daughter and answer her questions. She has frequent surgeries, and I do everything I can to
make it bearable. I asked staff at the hospital, our primary doctor, and several nurse friends for recommendations. We went to
meet the anesthesiologist who received the most endorsements,
and she's fabulous. We make sure the office always schedules
us with Dr. V. and we call the operating room the day before to
confirm it was done.*

Preparing your child

Most children cope best with surgery if you prepare them by explaining why the surgery is necessary and what it entails. The amount and type of information you give your child depends on his age and temperament. Using age-appropriate explanations to prepare your child will help him understand what is happening and reduce any fears or anxiety he may be feeling. Siblings also need to be prepared for the upcoming event (see Chapter 13, *Siblings*). Below are a few general guidelines for preparing your child, keeping in mind that each child is different and you know your child best.

- **Toddlers (ages 1–2).** The day before the surgery, give a simple explanation such as "The doctor is going to fix the owies in your ears." Give choices about what to pack and say that you'll be seeing the doctor in a hospital. Looking at a book about a visit to the hospital is very helpful (see the *Resources* section for suggestions).

- **Preschoolers (ages 3–5).** A day or two before the surgery, describe the type of surgery and when it will happen. Make sure your child knows why the surgery is necessary (e.g., "The doctor is going to fix your tonsils") because some children this age think surgery is a punishment for "being bad." Reassure your preschooler that you will stay with her in the hospital. Playing about the surgery helps (e.g., with dolls, toy doctors' kits) as does talking with a child life specialist and your pediatrician.

- **School-aged children (ages 6–12).** One or two weeks before the surgery, explain what it is, why it is necessary, and when it will happen. Together, read age-appropriate books or watch videos supplied by the doctor. When talking about the surgery, use terms your child will understand, be honest, and answer all questions. If you don't know the answer, tell your child you'll find out, and then do that.

- **Teens (ages 13–18).** Parents and teens should be partners in obtaining accurate information and making decisions about the surgery. Your teenager may be concerned about body image, privacy, or things that might affect her relationships with friends, so it is important to talk about these issues and feelings honestly. Encourage your teen to ask the doctors and nurses questions and talk over any concerns.

Your child likely will have questions about surgery that might not occur to you. You can read books about hospitals together to give your child a chance to ask questions (some suggestions are in the *Resources* section at the end of this book).

> *My daughter, Claire, has been hospitalized twice, for a tonsil-lectomy and to have tubes put in her ears. Before both surgeries, we took her to the grocery store to pick out Popsicles® and ice cream for when she came home. We went to the bookstore where she picked books to read and the movie rental store for movies. We also let her choose new sheets for her bed and new pajamas. All these things gave her some control over what was going to happen, as well as something exciting to look forward to after the surgery. It allowed us to explain that she would be sore and tired, but we could still have a fun time.*

It's a good idea to also explain anesthesia: your child will be given medicine that cause a special kind of sleep and, when she wakes up, the surgery will be over. Young children need to understand that sleep under anesthesia is not the same as regular sleep. Explain that she will not wake up during surgery and will not remember what happens.

Try to arrange a meeting between your child and members of the medical team, particularly the surgeon and anesthesiologist. The doctors and nurses on the team can answer questions and are less likely to frighten your child if their faces are familiar. See Chapter 3, *Preparing Your Child,* about taking a hospital tour and how child life specialists can help prepare your child for surgery. Many hospitals now have online tours and age-appropriate interactive activities to help prepare children for upcoming surgeries.

Young children also need to know that they will ride to surgery in a bed on wheels and, in the operating room, doctors and nurses will wear blue face masks and hair nets and outfits that look like blue pajamas. You can tell your child that, even though he has met the surgeon, it might be hard to identify him among the other blue-masked people.

Your doctor or surgeon can explain to your child what to expect after surgery: an IV, catheter, bandages, stitches, or the need for crutches or a wheelchair. Also, try to prepare your child for any pain. For example, her throat will hurt after her tonsils are removed or his belly may ache after a hernia operation. Most children can tolerate some discomfort, but they do better when prepared for it.

Other things to know before surgery:

- **Instructions for the night before.** Find out when your child must stop eating and drinking. For example, sometimes the instructions say do not eat or drink after midnight before the surgery. Scheduling the surgery for early morning can prevent hunger and thirst from becoming a problem for your youngster.

- **Prescriptions.** If you can get prescriptions for medications ahead of time, it may be easier for you to fill them before the surgery, rather than after.

- **Diet and exercise after surgery.** Ask whether there will be any restrictions on diet or exercise after the surgery. For example, if your child is having surgery of the mouth of throat, you might want to stock up on soft foods ahead of time.

> *After Claire had her tonsillectomy, she was feeling pretty good. A friend and her three children came to visit her at home that evening. The kids went out and played hard: swinging on the swings and running around. I should have known to keep her calmer and told them to go home much earlier. The visit really stressed her system and she was very ill for the next two days.*

The surgery

Some hospitals allow parents to be present when a child is sedated or anesthetized, others don't. Many parents feel strongly that they should be present until their child is safely sedated and also when their child wakes up. If you feel this way, talk about your wishes in the first meeting with the surgeon.

> *I told the staff that I needed to be with Christine when she was sedated and when she woke up. Parents going into the*

*recovery room was not standard practice, so the surgeon made
the arrangements well before the surgery. When they gave
Christine the pre-op meds, she got very goofy and giggly. She
smiled and waved to me as they pushed her gurney into the
operating room. After the surgery, I was the first thing she saw
when she opened her eyes.*

Your child may be frightened when an anesthesia mask is placed over
his face. Many anesthesiologists will give the child a choice of gas
flavorings to make the mask more acceptable. If you are present, you
can comfort your child by holding his hand, singing to him, telling
stories, or simply making sure he can see you until he closes his eyes.

As much as you'd like to, you cannot follow your child into surgery.
The wait may be difficult, but this is a good time to get a breath of
fresh air, eat something, make a telephone call, or take a quick break
from hospital routine. Your child will need you when she wakes up
and the more relaxed and comfortable you are, the better both of
you will feel.

The recovery room

Some hospitals allow parents into the recovery room, others do not.
Find out the hospital's policy and explain this to your child prior to
surgery so your child will know what to expect upon awakening.
Whether you meet your child in the recovery room or later, comfort
him any way you can: hold his hand, rock him, sing songs, play
music, watch TV, or read him a book.

*Charley was groggy after the surgery and very uncomfortable.
I told the nurse, and they gave him some pain medication and
then he smiled for the first time. We were in the recovery room
for a couple of hours before they moved him upstairs. He didn't
want to listen to music or look at books, so I climbed in the bed
and we just cuddled.*

If you are going home after the surgery, your child will stay in the
recovery room until the staff says she is awake enough to leave (e.g.,
when she can sip water or eat a Popsicle®). If your child is going to
stay in the hospital after surgery, he will be wheeled up to his room
after the recovery room staff says it's safe to go.

Going home

You may have to provide some medical care when your child comes home. If so, arrange to have the necessary medical equipment at home before your child leaves the hospital. Also try to make any special accommodations in advance, such as creating a sleeping area downstairs if your child won't be able to climb the stairs. If your hospital has a discharge planner or social worker, talk with her well before your child's discharge time, to make sure that you have all the information you need.

If your child needs nursing care, physical therapy, or other services at home, make sure the doctor writes that in the discharge papers. Some insurers refuse to pay for care after hospitalization unless there is a documented medical need.

Your family may need a few days or weeks to rest and recover before life returns to normal. Don't be afraid to tell family and friends that you need some down time for a few days after your child comes home. Hospitalization can be very stressful for families and everyone may benefit from time to decompress. However, if you like having family and friends around to pitch in and help or to keep your child company, let people know.

> After a long and tough hospitalization, 4-year-old Christine walked in the door, kissed her sister, kissed each dog, grabbed her blankie, wrapped herself in it, crawled up on the couch, let out a big sigh, and said "Finally, I'm home."

Chapter 9

Pain Management

"Pain is a thing that is glad to be forgotten."
— Robinson Jeffers

HOSPITALIZATION OFTEN RESULTS IN SOME amount of pain for children. Procedures such as blood draws, IV insertions, setting a bone, or getting stitches are common and painful events. The first few days after surgery can also be painful if adequate pain medication is not given. However, great strides have been made in preventing and treating pain in children.

The two primary methods to prevent pain during procedures are psychological (using the mind) and pharmacological (using medications). Medications—from mild to strong—are used during and after surgery to prevent or manage children's pain.

Psychological method

There is no fear greater than fear of the unknown. If children understand what is going to happen, where it will happen, who will be there, and what it will feel like, they will be better able to cope. Before any painful procedure, you can ask the hospital's child life specialist, psychologist, or nurse to discuss the upcoming procedure with your child.

- Explain each step in the procedure. Even if you think your child understands, ask him to tell you what he thinks will happen. Many parents are very surprised by their child's misconceptions.

- If possible, meet the person who will perform the procedure and let your child ask questions.

- Tour the room where the procedure will take place.

- See the instruments that will be used.

- Allow small children to play the procedure with dolls.

- Let older children observe a demonstration on a doll.
- Show adolescents videos that describe the procedure.
- Encourage discussion and answer all questions.

> Seven-year-old Tayler needed frequent blood draws to monitor
> the level of Dilantin® given for seizures. Before the first blood
> draw, we bought a new doll and poked her with needles. Then
> we went to the lab and met Barb—the technician. She told
> Tayler about her dogs (their pictures were on the walls). Barb
> and Taylor really connected. Barb showed her the needles and
> let Tayler watch some people have their blood drawn. Barb
> reassured her that, "I am very good and very fast at this."
> Tayler felt much better after the visit.

There's no substitute for good preparation to help your child get through a medical procedure. But you may also be able to use psychological techniques to lessen your child's pain during the procedure.

Imagery is an effective way to manage discomfort, but it requires practice before the procedure. Your child will visually focus on one object in the room, hold your hand, breathe deeply, and imagine a tranquil scene.

> I discovered my special place when I was 12, during a relax-
> ation session. My place is surrounded by sand and tall, fanning
> palm trees are everywhere. The sky is always clear; the sun
> shines bright. Each time I come to this place, I lie down to feel
> the gritty sand beneath me. Once in a while I get up and go
> looking for seashells. I feel the breeze going right through me,
> and I can smell the salt water. Whenever I feel sad or alone, or
> if I am in pain, I usually go jump in the water because it is a
> soothing place for me. I like to float in the water because it gives
> me a refreshing feeling that nobody can hurt me there.

You can use distraction techniques with children of all ages, but they should not be used as a substitute for preparation before the procedure or medication during the procedure (if needed). Colorful, moving objects will distract babies. Parents can distract preschoolers by showing picture books or videos, telling stories, singing songs, or blowing bubbles. Hugging a favorite stuffed animal comforts many youngsters. School-age children and teens can watch television or listen to music. Several institutions use interactive videos to help distract children or teens.

> *Our son has a chronic illness that requires daily shots. He is in charge of the process (which he often changes). Right now, the special Band-Aid® that looks like a tattoo needs to be open on the table; the appropriate site (left or right thigh) agreed upon, pinched, and alcohol-swabbed; a sibling holding one hand and he pinching an ear with the other; on the count of three the QUICK injection, followed as nearly instantaneously as possible by the Band-Aid®. No fear and no tears.*

In some hospitals, music therapists help decrease discomfort during procedures by using guided imagery or progressive muscle relaxation exercises while the children listen to music. Other therapies that are sometimes used to help deal with discomfort during medical treatments are relaxation, biofeedback, massage, and acupuncture.

Preventing pain during procedures

Most hospitals administer local anesthetic, temporary sedation, or general anesthesia prior to painful procedures (e.g., spinal tap). If these are not offered, you can request them. Discuss with your doctor and anesthesiologist which method will work best for your child.

The ideal pain relief drug for children should be easy to administer, have minimal and predictable effects, provide adequate pain relief, and last for a short time. Pain medication for procedures can be given by IV, on the skin, by mouth, and even by lollipop.

> *My son was in pediatric intensive care with a fractured skull from a bike accident. They had him sedated but I didn't think they were giving him adequate pain medication. He was unconscious but still crying. The nurse called the doctor but couldn't get the instructions changed. I asked her to note on the chart, "Parent demands to meet with doctor to discuss pain management." In the morning, in walked a new doctor who said, "Hello, my name is Dr. S., I have rewritten the orders to eliminate the sedation and increase his pain meds." Problem solved.*

Sedation and general anesthesia can result in complications. A board certified anesthesiologist should handle the sedation or anesthesia, and your child should be closely monitored until she is fully awake.

Reducing pain after trauma or surgery

Because trauma or surgery can cause moderate to severe pain, your child will be given pain medications by IV or mouth while recovering from the surgery in the hospital. If your child is in the intensive care unit after surgery, he may also receive sedatives along with pain relievers. Sedatives can decrease anxiety, induce sleep, and eliminate the memory of unpleasant events.

> Tucker was three when he had an emergency operation to repair an inguinal hernia. We were potty training him and after a session on the toilet trying to have a bowel movement he was in extreme pain. We took him to the emergency room and they discovered that part of his bowel was stuck in an abnormal opening in his abdominal wall. When he first woke up after surgery, he had no pain at all. However, after a few hours he got worse and worse. He was grumpy, wouldn't get up, and only wanted to watch his very favorite cartoon over and over again. At first we didn't realize it was pain, because he couldn't describe what was wrong, but after he got pain medication he was hard to keep still. The doctor told us that he would be back to his usual self in a couple of days, and he was, but it took a long time to get him to go back on the toilet.

Determining if your child is in pain

Infants, toddlers, school-aged children, and teenagers all show pain in different ways.

- Infants in pain move less. They may become irritable and cry frequently. Their appetites decrease. They may cry out if moved or touched. Parents know their infants well, and should advocate for appropriate medication if their infant is in pain.

- Preschoolers may become irritable, cry, or strike out if they are in pain. They may lose all interest in playing. Their breathing can become rapid and shallow. They might not be able to describe the pain in words, but may point to what hurts if asked, "Where is your owie?"

- School-aged children will be able to tell you when they are hurting. You can ask your child where it hurts and how much it hurts. Nurses should have sheets with a series of faces (from smiling to crying) that may help your child explain the amount of pain he is feeling. Some young children won't express pain because they fear that they will "get a shot." Take time beforehand to explain that they can get pain medicine through an IV line or by mouth and that the medicine will make them feel better, not worse.

- Teenagers react to pain like adults do. They may become angry, withdraw, have disrupted sleep and appetites, or become quiet and still. Any behavior changes should be investigated. Teens may not report pain for fear of taking drugs or becoming addicted. Reassure your teen that patients rarely become addicted to pain medication given for short periods of time in the hospital. Accurate, factual information about pain and pain control is crucial for adolescents.

Medications used to treat pain

Children's pain is typically treated with the same drugs used for adults. Mild pain may be treated with ibuprofen or acetaminophen (Tylenol®). Mild narcotics, such as codeine, are used for moderate pain. Severe pain—such as might be experienced the first few days after major surgery—can be effectively treated with one or more medications. These drugs can be given by mouth, by IV, in a suppository (most often given if a child has nausea or vomiting), or by injection (rare in children).

Pain medication should decrease or eliminate your child's pain. If the prescribed medications are not curbing your child's pain, or your child is very nauseated, tell the nurse and doctor. Most hospitals have a "pain team" of specialists in pain control. Ask for a consultation with this team if your child's pain is not well managed.

If your doctor prescribes pain medications to be taken after your child is discharged, pick up the prescription at the hospital's pharmacy or your local pharmacy on the way home. Be sure to follow the doctor's directions to keep a constant level of medication in your child's body. If you wait until your child is in severe pain before giving the medication, it will take a higher dose and will take longer for your child to become comfortable again. Make sure to store all medications away from children or pets.

Chapter 10

Family and Friends:
What to Say

"Shared joy is double joy,
shared sorrow is half sorrow."
— Swedish proverb

AN ILLNESS OR INJURY SERIOUS ENOUGH to require hospitalization creates a ripple effect, first touching the immediate family, then extended family, friends, coworkers, schoolmates, and faith communities. Parents will find that family members and friends help them in extraordinary ways. But sometimes, people who could provide the greatest support may become sources of added stress.

Notifying family and friends

If your child goes to the hospital for a routine procedure or minor injury, you probably won't have to communicate with anyone outside the immediate family. When the illness or injury is serious, notifying family and friends becomes a painful necessity.

One easy way to tell family and friends is to delegate one person to do the job. Calling one relative, neighbor, or close friend prevents numerous conversations about the illness or injury. Most parents are at their child's bedside and want to avoid more emotional upheaval, especially in front of their child.

> *The first three days in the hospital after my daughter was diagnosed with a serious disease, I spent much of my time crying on the phone when talking to friends and relatives. Then I realized how frightening this must be to my two-year-old. So I just stopped talking on my cell phone. Now, each time Jennifer is hospitalized, I call one friend and have her spread the news, then I concentrate on my daughter.*

You can tell a trusted family member friend exactly what information you want him or her to pass on and, most importantly, whether you would welcome visits, phone calls, or cards. If you want visitors, for example, let people know when visiting hours are and whether there are any restrictions set by the hospital (or by you or your child) about who can come and for how long.

Parents usually find that relatives' and friends' emotions will mirror their own: shock, fear, worry, helplessness. Since most loved ones want to help but don't know what to do or say, they welcome cues about what might help.

Sometimes, especially when an illness or injury is severe, parents must take extra steps to keep family members and friends informed and involved.

- Encourage all members of the family to keep in touch through visits, calls, email, or social media.

- Call if you don't hear from family members or close friends. Often silence means they don't know what to do or say.

- Tell family members and friends when your child is too sick or too fatigued for company. When visits are welcome, make them brief and cheerful.

What to say

Many people feel awkward and tongue-tied in the presence of families with an injured or ill child, particularly if the injury or illness is severe. Kind words are always welcome and a specific offer of help can be accepted or graciously declined. Here are a few suggestions of helpful things to say.

- "I am so sorry" (follow with a big hug).

- "Our family would like to mow the lawn, weed the flower beds, and rake the leaves. Is this weekend a good time?"

- "We want to clean your house for you once a week. What day would be convenient?"

- "Would it help if we took care of your dog (or cat, or bird)? We would love to do it."

- "The church (or synagogue or mosque) is setting up a system to deliver meals to your house. When is the best time to drop them off?"

- "I will take care of Joanie whenever you need to take Jimmy to the hospital. Call us any time, day or night, and we will come pick her up."

> *Many well-wishing friends always said, "Let me know what I can do." I wish they had just "done," instead of asking for direction. It took too much energy to decide, call them, and make arrangements. I wish someone would have said, "I'll bring dinner," or "I'll baby-sit Sunday afternoon so you and your husband can go out to lunch together."*

Things that do not help

Well-meaning people sometimes say hurtful things to parents of sick or injured children. If you are a family member or friend of a parent with a hospitalized child, please do not say any of the following:

- "God only gives people what they can handle." Some people cannot handle the stress related to their child's illness or injury.

- "I know just how you feel." Unless you have a child in a similar situation, you simply don't know.

- "You are so brave," or "You are so strong." Parents of very sick children are not heroes; they are ordinary people struggling with extraordinary stress.

Parents also make the following suggestions of things to avoid doing:

- Do not make personal comments in front of the child: "He's lost so much weight," or "She's so pale."

- Do not do things that require the parent to support you (for example, call up repeatedly, crying).

- Especially if treatments are lengthy, do not talk continually about the illness. Some normal conversations are welcome.

Most parents welcome stories of other children you know who had a similar condition and are doing fine.

Using technology to keep in touch

After the initial contacts have been made, the people in your life will be eager for updates, and many families use technology to keep in touch. Many hospitals now have free wireless internet access (Wi-Fi) in the room, in the parents' lounge, or in a communal room. Some internet service providers offer their own Wi-Fi adapters that can be plugged into a laptop to provide access anywhere there is cell phone service. Smartphones and other personal data devices also have internet access.

Once connected to the internet, many options exist for keeping in touch, including Facebook®, Twitter®, and blogs. Some parents establish an email group and send regular updates to the list. If your child has a lengthy hospitalization, one easy way to communicate with your friends and family is to use CaringBridge (*www.caringbridge. org*), which provides free websites to families and friends of seriously ill individuals. Its templates make it easy to set up an attractive site, and the software allows you to add text and photos. Parents, siblings, or the sick child can create journal entries that track the progress of treatment and discuss fears, inspirations, hopes, or needs. There is a guest book where well-wishers can post words of love and encouragement. Finally, you can make the site as public or private as you wish and link your site to other places, such as a blog or Facebook® page.

Chapter 11

Family and Friends: How to Help

"We can do no great things—only small things with great love."

— Mother Theresa

A CHILD'S SERIOUS SICKNESS OR INJURY can overwhelm a family—affecting finances, emotions, and time with siblings. Help from friends and relatives is a crucial part of the family's ability to cope with the disruption in their lives.

Many relatives and friends genuinely want to help, but don't know how. The following sections describe helpful things you can do for a family with a child in the hospital. Although some of the suggestions listed are most appropriate when dealing with lengthy illnesses or recoveries, they may give you some good ideas for any hospitalization.

Help at the hospital

Friends and family members can find many ways to make a child's hospital experience more bearable.

- Send balloon bouquets, funny cards, posters, toys, or humorous books. A cheerful hospital room really boosts a child's spirits.

- Send funny videotapes or arrive with a good joke. Laughter helps heal the mind and body.

- Bring toys, puzzles, games, picture books, coloring books, age-appropriate computer games, and crafts.

- Bring a basket of meals or snacks.

- Offer to give parents a break from the hospital room. A walk outside, shopping trip, haircut, or a long shower can be very refreshing.

- Donate frequent flyer miles to distant family members who have the time—but not the money—to help, if the treatment or illness is lengthy or severe.

- Donate blood. Your blood won't necessarily be used for the injured child, but will replenish the general supply.

> One of the nicest things that friends did was to bring a huge picnic basket full of food to the hospital. We spread a blanket on the floor, Erica crawled out of bed, and the entire family sat down together and ate. Most people don't realize how expensive it is to have to eat every meal at the hospital cafeteria, so the picnic was not only fun, but helped us save a few dollars.

Household

Parents of sick or injured children often don't have time to do daily chores. Friends and family can help with these routine tasks. Even when the illness or injury is not too severe, a home-cooked meal or a bag of small toys can express love and provide comfort. Household tasks that family members of friends can do are:

- Provide meals

- Take care of pets or livestock

- Mow grass, shovel snow, rake leaves, weed gardens

- Clean house

- Grocery shop (especially when the family is due home from the hospital)

- Do laundry

- Provide a place to stay near the hospital

> Friends from home sent boxes of art supplies to us when the whole family spent those first ten weeks in the Ronald McDonald House far from home. They sent scissors, paints,

paper, colored pens. It was a great help for Carrie Beth and her two sisters. One friend even sent an Easter package with straw hats for each girl, and flowers, ribbons, and glue to decorate them with.

Siblings

Siblings of hospitalized children need lots of love, attention, and care. Friends and family can help when parents are overwhelmed.

- Baby-sit whenever parents go to doctor's appointments, the emergency room, or during a prolonged hospital stay.

- When parents are home with a sick child, take siblings to a park, sports event, or movie.

- Invite siblings over for meals.

- If you bring a gift for the sick child, bring something for the siblings.

- Offer to help siblings with homework.

- Drive siblings to lessons, games, or school.

- Listen to siblings when they need to talk.

Psychological support

Parents of a sick or injured child can feel overwhelmed, frightened, and exhausted. They need practical and emotional help from family and friends.

- Call frequently. Be open to listening if parents want to talk about their feelings.

- Call to talk about topics other than the child's illness or injury.

- Stay in the hospital with the sick child if parents have to work.

- Drive parent and child to the hospital.

- Buy books (humorous or uplifting ones) for family members if they are readers.

- Baby-sit the sick child so parents can go out to eat, exercise, take a walk, or just get out of the hospital.

- Give lots of hugs.

> *Word got around my parents' hometown, and I received cards from many high school acquaintances, who still cared enough to call or write and say we're praying for you, please let us know how things are going. It was so neat to get so many cards out of the blue that said, "I'm thinking about you."*

Financial support

Helping a family keep track of finances while a child is sick or injured can be a great gift. Even fully insured families can spend up to twenty-five percent of their income on copayments, travel, motels, meals, and other uncovered items when a child has a long-term, serious illness or injury. Uninsured or underinsured families can lose their savings, or even their house. Friends and family can find many ways to help.

- Start a support fund.

- Share leave. The federal government and some companies have leave banks that permit people who are ill or taking care of someone who is ill to use coworkers' leave so they won't lose pay.

- Collect money by organizing a bake sale, dance, or raffle.

- Give the family gift certificates from restaurants that deliver meals.

- Handle hospital bills. Keeping track of medical bills can be time-consuming, frustrating, and exhausting. If you are a close relative or friend, you could offer to review, organize, and file (or enter into a computer) the voluminous paperwork. Making calls and writing letters about contested claims or billing errors can be very helpful.

> *My husband's coworkers didn't collect money, they did something even more valuable. They donated sick leave hours, so that he was able to be at the hospital frequently during those first few months without losing a paycheck.*

Help from schoolmates

Classmates and friends can be a huge help to sick or injured children by giving them support and encouragement and helping them feel connected.

- Encourage visits (if appropriate), cards, and phone calls from classmates.

- Make sure the visiting children are prepared for what they will see at the hospital. Tell their parents, "Joey will have a tube in his nose," or "Carrie's skin will be puffy."

- Ask the teacher to send the school newspaper and other news along with assignments.

- Classmates can sign a brightly colored banner to send to the hospital.

- The teacher or principal can put the entire class on a speaker-phone to chat with their classmate.

> Brent's kindergarten class sent a packet containing a picture drawn for him by each child in the class. They also made him a book. Another time they sent him a letter written on huge poster board. He couldn't wait to get back to school.

Religious support

Religious communities can be sources of both spiritual and practical help.

- Arrange for the pastor, rabbi, or church members to visit the hospital, if the family wants

- Arrange prayer services for the sick child

- Ask the child's religious education class to send pictures, posters, letters, balloons, or tapes to the sick or injured child

> The day our son was diagnosed, we raced next door to ask our wonderful neighbors to take care of our dog. The news of his diagnosis quickly spread, and we found out later that five neighborhood families gathered that very night to pray for Brent.

Chapter 12

Feelings and Behavior

"Example is not the main thing in influencing others—it is the only thing."

— Albert Schweitzer

UNDER THE BEST OF CIRCUMSTANCES, child rearing is a daunting task. When parenting is complicated by a child's serious illness or sudden hospitalization, communication within the family may suffer. Sharing feelings and managing changes in behavior will help keep the family on an even keel.

Feelings

Children can be overcome with feelings when they are sick or hurt. At varying times and to varying degrees, children and teens may feel fearful, angry, resentful, powerless, violated, lonely, weird, inferior, incompetent, betrayed. All these feelings, if left unresolved, create stress. Children need to learn ways to deal with these feelings to prevent acting out (by throwing tantrums, for example) or acting in (becoming depressed or withdrawn).

Good communication is the first step toward helping your family cope with the feelings and changes brought about by illness or injury.

- **Honesty.** Above all, children must be able to trust their parents. They can face almost anything when they know their parents will be at their side. Trust requires honesty. For children to feel secure, they must know they can depend on their parents to tell them the truth, be it good news or bad.

  I have found that as my children's understanding of the illness deepens, they come back with more questions, needing more detailed answers. So, my motto is, be honest but don't scare them. If you say everything is okay but you are crying, they know something is wrong, and that they can't trust you to tell the truth.

- **Listening.** Time is one of the greatest gifts you can give your children. Children need you to really focus on what they are saying. Listen to their words and the feelings behind them, and stop to think before responding.

- **Touching.** Hospitalized children need lots of back rubs and hugs. Children, sick or well, need frequent contact with parents. Be sure your kids know you have an unlimited supply of hugs.

> When my daughter was seven, three years after her treatment ended, I realized how important it is to keep listening. She was complaining about a hangnail so I told her I would cut it. She yelled I would hurt her. I asked, "When have I ever hurt you?" She said, "In the hospital." I sat down and rocked her in my arms, explained what had happened in the hospital during her treatment, why we had to bring her, and how we felt about it. I asked how she felt about being there. We cleared the air that day, and I expect we will need to talk about it many more times. Then she held out her hand so that I could cut her hangnail.

Some parents like to keep a list of reminders about how manage strong feelings when both children and parents are stressed.

- Model the type of behavior you desire. If you talk respectfully and take timeouts when angry, your child will learn to do likewise. If you scream and hit, that is how your child will handle his anger.

- Teach your child to talk about her feelings.

- Distinguish between having feelings (always okay) and acting on feelings in destructive or hurtful ways (not okay).

- Listen to your child with understanding and empathy.

- Be honest and admit your mistakes.

- Help your child examine why he is behaving as he is.

- Have clear rules and consequences.

- Discuss acceptable outlets for anger.

- Give frequent reassurances of your love.

- Provide lots of hugs and physical affection.

- Compliment your child for good behavior.

- Recognize that disturbing behaviors can result from stress, pain, and drugs.

- Remember that with lots of structure, love, and time, problems will become more manageable.

Behavior changes

Some children, due to temperament and upbringing, are blessed with good coping abilities. They understand what is needed to cope and they find ways to manage. Many parents express great admiration for their child's strength and grace in the face of adversity. It is common, however, for family members to respond to the illness in the family with changes in feelings and behavior.

- **Anger.** Parents often respond to illness or injury with anger. So do children. Children rage at their pain and at their parents for bringing them to the hospital to be hurt. Sick or injured children have good reasons to be angry.

- **Problems sleeping.** Children often express stress by feeling unable to sleep alone or by having nightmares. Some parents allow the child to sleep with them, while others try soothing bedtime rituals or seek therapy.

- **Tantrums.** Healthy children have tantrums when they are overwhelmed by their feelings. So do sick or injured children. You can often predict tantrums by paying close attention to what triggers the outburst. This can help you prevent tantrums by avoiding situations that overload your child.

> At one point Caitlin had overeaten her beloved French fries and had a "worse than agony case of gas," as she described it. She spent the evening howling and really created a stir on the pediatric floor. She had a classic tantrum. I went in to take a shower and, when I returned to her room, there was a note taped to her door apologizing to all the people on the floor for her screaming attack.

- **Withdrawal.** Some children withdraw rather than blow up in anger. Like denial, withdrawal can temporarily help a child come to grips with strong feelings. However, too much withdrawal can be a sign of depression or psychological trauma. Parents or counselors can gently encourage withdrawn children to express their feelings.

> In the first few days of hospitalization, my three-year-old daughter stopped interacting with everyone. She lay on the bed with her face turned to the wall. She wouldn't talk, make eye contact, or respond in any way. She would totally ignore us if we tried to comfort her with stories, songs, or hugs. She tuned us out. We asked for help and a psychiatric nurse worked with her for two hours. We don't know what she did, but when we came back in, our daughter was sitting up in bed painting her fingernails.

- **Regression.** Many parents worry if children regress to using a special comfort object when they are sick or hurt. Many young children return to using a bottle, or cling to a favorite toy or blanket. Allow your child to use whatever he can to find comfort. The behaviors usually stop when the child starts feeling better or when treatment ends.

> Our son has a serious condition that has required years of difficult treatments. He is either very defiant or an absolute angel. Sometimes he argues about every single thing. I think it is because he has had so little control in his life. I have clear rules, am very firm, and put my foot down. But I also try to choose my battles wisely, so that we can have good times, too. My husband reminds me that if he wasn't this type of tough kid, he wouldn't have made it through the years of treatment, including so many setbacks.

Communication and discipline

Short-term hospitalizations or outpatient surgeries may create only minor disruptions in your family's routines. However, long-term treatments or lengthy hospitalization increases the need for consistent rules. Parents of children with difficult or long-term illnesses share the following techniques to help improve communication and maintain discipline within the family.

- Make sure all the children clearly understand the family rules. Stressed children feel safer in homes with structured, predictable routines.

- Enforce family rules consistently. Make sure all caregivers know the rules.

- Give kids some power. Offer choices and, as appropriate, let them control some aspects of their lives and medical treatment.

  All these interns at the teaching hospital came in and said, "Can we listen to David's heart?" He sat up and said, "You ask me." All the females got to listen and none of the males. He wanted to control who listened to his heart and he only picked the female interns.

- Take charge of incoming gifts. Too many gifts can make an ill child worry ("If I'm getting all of these great presents, things must be really bad"). Gifts also make siblings jealous. Be specific if you want people not to bring gifts, or if you want gifts for each child, not just the sick one. When a child has an illness or injury that requires long-term care, some parents gather the gifts and hand them out at regular intervals throughout treatment.

- Discuss acceptable ways to physically release anger. Children can ride a bike, run around the house, swing, play basketball or soccer, pound nails into wood, mold clay, punch pillows, yell, take a shower or bath, or draw angry pictures.

- Teach your child to use words to express her anger, for example, "It makes me furious when you do that," or, "I am so mad I feel like screaming at you." Expressing anger verbally is a valuable life skill to master.

- Treat the sick or hurt child as normally as possible.

- Try to determine whether the illness or injury is aggravating a pre-existing problem. If so, treat the problem, not the symptoms.

- Find a professional counselor who specializes in children whenever you are concerned about your child's behavior. Mental health professionals know how to resolve problems—give them a chance to help you.

- Teach children relaxation or visualization skills to help them cope with their feelings.

- If your child likes to draw, paint, knit, do collages, or other artwork, encourage it. Art is soothing and therapeutic. It allows the child a positive outlet for feelings and creativity. Making something beautiful really helps raise children's spirits.

- Allow your child to be totally in charge of his art. Do not make suggestions or criticize (by saying, "stay inside the lines," or, "skies need to be blue not orange"). Rather, encourage him and praise his efforts. Display the artwork in your home or your child's hospital room. Listen carefully if your child offers an explanation of the art, but do not pry if it is private. Being supportive will allow your child to explore ways to soothe himself and clarify his feelings.

  > Jody was continually working on art projects when he was in the bone marrow transplant unit. We kept him supplied with a fishing box full of materials, and he glued and taped and constructed all sorts of sculptures. He did beautiful drawings full of color, and every person he drew always had hands shaped like hearts. If we asked him what he was making, he always answered, "I'll show you when I'm done."

- Help your child start and keep a journal to draw in and to record feelings, events, and visits. This can become an important emotional outlet.

- Have reasonable expectations. If you are expecting a sick four-year-old to act like a healthy six-year-old, or a teenager to act like an adult, you are setting up your child to fail.

- Give children time to process the experience of illness, hospitalization, and treatment. Many children talk about their hospital experience for months after returning home or recreate it when they play.

Chapter 13
Siblings

*"Sometimes being a brother is
even better than being a superhero."*

— Marc Brown

A CHILD'S HOSPITALIZATION TOUCHES all members of the family, especially siblings. Even a short-term hospital stay can disrupt a sibling's sense of security and routine. An illness or injury in the family can create an array of conflicting emotions in siblings. They worry about their ill brother or sister yet might resent the turmoil in their family. They may feel jealous if gifts and attention are showered on the sick child and then feel guilty for having these emotions.

Many problems can be prevented by preparing siblings just like you do the child who will be hospitalized. Reading books together and taking them on the hospital tour will help give them a better understanding of why their brother or sister needs to go to the hospital. These activities also can spur discussion and give you a chance to clear up any misconceptions or worries your healthy children have.

Emotional responses

A child's illness or injury can deeply upset her brothers and sisters. If the injury is serious or the illness prolonged, parents may have little time or energy to focus on the siblings. Siblings may be flooded with anger and concern, jealousy and love. If you recognize that these emotions are normal, you will be better able to help your children talk about and cope with their strong feelings. Some emotions the siblings may experience include:

- **Concern.** Children really worry about a sick brother or sister. It is hard for them to watch someone they love be hurt by an injury, surgery, or treatment for an illness. It is hard to feel so healthy and full of energy when your brother or sister has to stay in the hospital.

- **Fear.** Even if a brother or sister is injured or suffering from a non-communicable illness, young siblings may fear that they, their parents, or friends can "catch it." An illness or injury can also change a child's view that the world is a safe place. Depending on their age, siblings may worry that their brother or sister will get sicker. Fear of other things may emerge: fear of being hit by a car, fear of dogs, fear of strangers. Many fears can be quieted by accurate and age-appropriate explanations from parents or medical staff.

  > My older daughter spent a lot of time in the hospital. Her younger sister (three years old) vacillated between fear of catching her sister's illness and wishing she was ill so that she would get the gifts and attention ("I want to get sick and go to the hospital with mommy"). She developed many fears and had frequent nightmares. We did lots of medical play which seemed to help her.

- **Guilt.** Young children are egocentric; they believe the world revolves around them. It is logical for them to feel that they caused the illness or injury. You should try to dispel this notion right away. Children should be told that sickness and injury just happen, and no one in the family causes them.

- **Jealousy.** Despite feeling concerned for an ill brother or sister, siblings may also feel jealous. In the case of a serious injury or illness, presents and cards flood in for the sick child, mom and dad stay at the hospital with the sick child, and most conversations revolve around the sick child. When the siblings go out to play, the neighbors ask about the sick child. At school, teachers are concerned about the sick child. Is it any wonder that they feel jealous?

  > My fifteen-year-old daughter has severe endometriosis. It has required six surgeries and many emergency room visits. Because it's a disease that you can't see, her younger brother has a hard time accepting it. He says things like, "You're with her all the time," and, "She's just faking being sick." I realized that we needed to explain the situation again and also make special time for him. We needed to give him plenty of love and support, too.

- **Abandonment.** If all of your attention is focused on your ill child, your other children may feel isolated and resentful. Even when you make a conscious effort not to be preoccupied with their ill brother or sister, siblings often believe that they are not getting their fair share of attention, and may feel rejected.

  One day when my four-year-old son was in day care, we had to unexpectedly bring Erica in for emergency surgery on a septic hip. I called day care and said that I couldn't pick up Daniel by closing time. The teacher said, "No problem, I'll take him home for dinner." When we picked Daniel up that evening, he was very withdrawn. Later, he exclaimed, "All the mommies came. Then teacher turned out the lights, and you didn't come to get me," and he burst into tears. In hindsight, one of us should have gone to bring him to the hospital to sit with us. It was tense there, but at least he would have been with us.

- **Anger.** If siblings' lives are in turmoil, they may feel a need to blame someone. It's natural for them to think that if their brother didn't get sick, life would be back to normal. When the illness or injury is severe, questions such as, "Why did this happen to us?" or, "Why can't things be the way they used to be?" are common. Children's anger may be directed at their sick brother, their parents, relatives, friends, or the doctor. The anger may have many triggers, such as being left with baby-sitters, unequal application of family rules, or additional responsibilities at home. Because each member of the family may have frayed nerves, angry outbursts can occur.

- **Worry.** Children have vivid imaginations, especially when they are fueled by disrupted households and whispered conversations between parents. Frequent age-appropriate explanations can help children better understand what happens at the hospital, but nothing is as powerful as a visit. The effectiveness of a visit will depend on your child's age and temperament, but many parents say bringing the siblings along helps everyone. The sibling gains an accurate understanding of hospital procedures, the sick child is comforted by the presence of the sibling, and parents get to spend time with all their children.

I am the first of four children and the only girl. When I was diagnosed with leukemia at the age of fourteen, it affected all our lives. My brother Wes was thirteen, Matthew was four and Erik was two. They and my parents were my support system. Wes was my support at home and school. He stuck up for me and kept an eye on me. Matt and Erik would accompany my mom and me to treatments and hold my hand. If one of them wasn't with me when I went in, the nurses would ask where they were. These little boys made it easier for me to be brave.

- **Concern about parents.** Parents focused on helping their sick child get through an illness or injury often are not aware of their healthy children's strong feelings. They sometimes assume that children understand that they are loved, and would get the same attention if they were sick or injured. But siblings often do not share their feelings of anger, jealousy, or worry because they do not want to place additional burdens on their parents. It is all too common to hear siblings say, "I have to be the strong one. I don't want to cause my parents any more pain." But burdens are lighter if shared, and parents should try to encourage all their children to talk about how they are feeling.

Helping siblings cope

Being available to listen, to say, "I hear how painful this is for you," or, "You sound scared. I am, too," makes siblings feel they are still valued members of the family and, even though their sick or injured brother or sister is absorbing the lion's share of parents' time and care, they are still cherished. You can help siblings of a sick or injured child by keeping them involved, making sure they know they are loved, and addressing any problems that develop.

- Make sure that all the children clearly understand the nature of the illness or injury. If an illness is contagious, ask your doctor about special precautions and explain these to the whole family.

  I'm fifteen now. Looking back at my brother's long illness, the parts I hated the most were: not understanding what was being done to him, answering endless worried phone calls, and hearing the answers to my own questions when my parents talked to other people.

- Try to spend time individually with each sibling (e.g., take a trip, see a movie, or ride bicycles together).

- Include siblings in decision-making. Let them choose how to parcel out extra chores or plan a schedule for parent time with each child.

- Alert siblings' teachers about the stress at home. Many children respond to worries about a serious illness or injury by developing behavioral or academic problems at school. It helps to communicate frequently with siblings' teachers and try to stay abreast of any developing problems.

- Encourage a close relationship between an adult relative or friend and your other children. Having someone special around when parents are absent can prevent problems and help your child feel cared for and loved.

- Expect siblings to develop some strong feelings or behavioral problems if your child's illness or injury is long-term. This is normal.

- Give lots of hugs and kisses.

> Kim's hospitalizations were very hard on five-year-old Kelly.
> My parents kept Kelly during the week, so this helped a lot.
> My husband would pick her up after work. I remember being
> at the hospital all week long, then my husband would come on
> the weekends and I would go home and do things with Kelly.
> We would go out to eat, or go roller-skating. I really missed her
> and it was just so hard on everyone. I remember being so tired,
> but I feel that you need to spend time with all of your children
> because they need you also.

Chapter 14

Long-Term Illness
or Injury

*"Life can only be understood backwards;
however it must be lived forwards"*
— Søren Kierkegaard

AFTER A SHORT-TERM ILLNESS OR INJURY, most families return to normal routines quickly. But when the hospitalization lasts for weeks or months, family life can be very disrupted. This chapter contains some suggestions for dealing with the difficulties that sometimes accompany long-term illness or injury.

Taking care of yourself

You can run yourselves ragged when your child is in the hospital for a long time. Try to find one or two ways to stay healthy and feel balanced. Parents who have walked this road before you share the following ideas:

- Try to eat, sleep, and get a few minutes of exercise every day.

- Take turns staying with your child at night. If the hospital is far from home, you could rent a hotel room nearby, stay in a Ronald McDonald House or hospital hospitality house, or borrow a mobile home or trailer to park at the hospital. A refuge from the noise and smells of a hospital can be a welcome, and needed, relief.

> *Whenever Brent was in the hospital, we both wanted to be there. During his second extended stay in the hospital, we both let go a little, and we each took turns sleeping at the Ronald McDonald House. That way, we each got a decent night's sleep (or some sleep) every other night.*

- Ask a favorite aunt, uncle, or grandparent to spend nights at the hospital occasionally so both parents can go home to sleep. This can be especially comforting for siblings.

- Find ways to share your feelings about what is happening. You can talk with your spouse, another parent at the hospital, a friend, a family member, the hospital chaplain, or a counselor.

Work

In families with two parents, they must decide what to do about their jobs when facing a long-term hospitalization of their child. If you can, use all available sick leave and vacation days before you decide whether one parent should leave a job. The Family and Medical Leave Act (FMLA) protects job security of workers in large companies (50+ employees within a 75-mile radius) who must take a leave of absence for medical reasons, including caring for a seriously ill child, recovering from a medical condition, giving birth, or adopting a child. You can consult your employee handbook or director of human resources about whether your company is covered by this law.

Marriage

A child's life-threatening illness or injury can create enormous pressures in a marriage. Couples can be separated for long periods of time, emotions are high, and coping styles and skills may differ. Working together to handle the situation can help immensely. Parents shared the following suggestions:

- Share medical decisions

> My husband and I shared decision-making by keeping a joint medical journal. The days that my husband stayed at the hospital, he would write down all medicines given, side effects, fever, vital signs, food consumed, sleep patterns, and any questions that needed to be asked at the next rounds. This way, I knew exactly what had been happening. Decisions were made as we traded shifts at our son's bedside.

- Take turns staying in the hospital with your ill child

- Share responsibility for home care

- Make spending time together a priority, even if it is only thirty minutes a day for coffee in the hospital cafeteria

- Accept differences in coping styles

Marriages with existing troubles usually are most strained by caring for a gravely ill child. If serious conflicts develop, don't hesitate to seek outside help.

> My husband and I went to counseling to try to work out a way to split up the child rearing and household duties because I was overwhelmed and resenting it. It helped, but the best thing that came out of it was that I kept seeing the counselor by myself. I received a lot of very helpful, practical advice on the many behavior problems my son developed. My son wanted to go to a "feelings doctor" too. So we arranged that and he had an objective, safe person to talk things over with.

Divorced parents

Parents who were separated or divorced prior to their child's injury or illness face additional difficulties. They will have to work together to help their child.

- Agree to set aside differences for the duration of the crisis

- Focus on communication

- Make agreements and abide by them

- Go to mediation if conflicts cannot be resolved

Anything divorced parents can do to prevent or minimize stress will help all of their children.

Parents' reactions

Most parents experience a range of emotional and physical reactions to their child's serious illness or injury. Over time, many parents find unexpected reserves of strength and ask for help from their friends and family when they need it. They realize that family members' needs change during stressful times and they alter their expectations and parenting accordingly. But, it isn't easy. Following are common reactions to a child's serious illness or injury.

- **Illness.** Parents watching over children in the hospital often fail to eat and sleep. They become so focused on their child's health that they neglect their own. Plus, hospitals are full of germs. So it's not surprising that parents of children in the hospital often become ill themselves.

  > I lost thirty-five pounds in the first six weeks of my son's hospitalization. I had almost constant diarrhea and vomited frequently. After that first six weeks, I was able to worry less, eat more, and even laugh occasionally.

- **Confusion and numbness.** When a child is injured or very ill, parents often experience shock, followed by confusion and numbness. This is a normal reaction: the mind tries to block out painful information. The confusion will pass, but parents may need to take extra time to jot down information that they normally wouldn't have trouble remembering.

- **Feelings of helplessness.** A hospital has a routine of its own: every staff member has defined tasks and clear duties, but parents may feel helpless. Many parents say they feel more powerful when they establish a new routine and begin helping their child cope.

- **Anger.** Anger is a typical response to a child's serious illness or injury. Sometimes parents vent their anger on hospital staff or their family and friends. To cope with anger, parents should learn healthy ways to manage feelings, such as talking with friends, exercising, writing in a journal, or seeking counseling.

- **Sadness and grief.** Even when the child is expected to recover fully, parents may experience sadness and grief about their child's trauma. This is normal.

- **Hope.** Hope is the belief in a better tomorrow. It sustains the will to live and gives the strength to endure each trial. Cultivating a hopeful attitude will help you cope with your child's extended hospitalization—one day at a time.

I'm a controlled person. My four-year-old needed me to show I was upset, too. One day, after a blood draw, she yelled at me all the way to the car saying, "You just want them to hurt me; you don't love me; why do you take me to get hurt?" I sat in the car and burst into tears. I told her bringing her to the hospital so many times was the hardest thing I'd ever done. That I wished it was me who was sick, not her. That I loved her so much and wanted to protect her from hurt, but I couldn't. I told her that she would get better, but we just had to get through the hard treatments. She looked at me, patted me on the arm, and said, "It's okay now, Mom, let's just go home."

Behavior changes under extreme stress

When a child is very ill or seriously injured, parents can experience physical, emotional, financial, and spiritual stress. The crisis can result in difficult feelings and behaviors.

- **Dishonesty.** Children feel safe when their parents are honest with them. If parents keep secrets from children, or try to protect them from bad news, they feel isolated and fearful. A child might think, "If Mom and Dad won't tell me, it must be really bad," or, "Mom won't talk about it. I guess there's nobody that I can tell about how scared I am."

- **Denial.** Denial is a type of unconscious dishonesty. This occurs when parents say, "Everything will be just fine," or, "It won't hurt a bit." This type of pretending increases the distance between child and parent, leaving the child with no support. However horrible the truth, it seldom is as terrifying as a half-truth upon which a child's imagination builds.

- **Depression.** Depression can develop in parents of seriously hurt or sick children. Parents should seek professional help if they regularly experience any of the following symptoms: changes in sleeping patterns (sleeping too much, waking up frequently during the night), appetite disturbances (eating too little or too much), fatigue, panic attacks, inability to experience pleasure, feelings of sadness and despair, poor concentration, social withdrawal, feelings of worthlessness, suicidal thoughts, and drug or alcohol abuse. Depression can be treated with counseling, medication, or both.

- **Loss of temper.** All parents lose their tempers sometimes. They lose their tempers with spouses, healthy children, pets, even strangers. But anger can be especially painful when the target is a sick child. If stressed, parents can give themselves a ten-minute quiet time in private to regroup. If, despite their best efforts, parents find they are too stressed to control their tempers, a professional counselor can help them explore new ways of coping.

> I had always taught my children that feeling angry sometimes was normal, but we had to make good choices about what to do with it. Hitting other people or breaking things was a bad choice; punching pillows or running around outside were good choices. But, as with everything else, they learned the most from watching how I handled my anger, and during the hard months of treatment my temper was short. When I found myself thinking of hitting them, I'd say, in a very loud voice, "I'm afraid I'm going to hurt somebody so I'm going in my room for a time-out." If my husband was home, I'd take a warm shower to calm down; if he wasn't, I'd just lock myself in my bedroom, sit on the bed, and take as many deep breaths as it took to calm down.

- **Unequal application of household rules.** Parents guarantee family problems if the ill child enjoys favored status while the siblings must do extra chores. It is hard to know when to insist that a child with a long-term illness or injury resume making his bed or setting the table, but it must be done. Siblings should know from the very beginning that any child in the family, if sick, will be excused from chores, but must start again when he is able.

- **Overindulgence.** Parents often overindulge sick or injured children.

> When my daughter became very sick, I bought her everything that I saw that was pretty and lovely. I kept thinking that, if she died, she would die happy because she'd be surrounded by all these beautiful things. Even when I couldn't really afford it, I kept buying. I realize now that I was doing it to make me feel better, not her. She needed cuddling and loving, not clothes and dolls.

- **Overprotection.** Parents should ask the doctor what changes in physical activity are necessary for safety and not impose restrictions that go beyond this. Letting children become involved in sports or neighborhood play may be difficult, but it helps them feel better as well as develop friendships.

Chapter 15
School

"Education is an ornament in prosperity
and a refuge in adversity."
— Aristotle

Sick or injured children often experience disruptions in their education. These can range from a few missed lessons to long-term absences caused by repeated hospitalizations or side effects from medication.

Returning to school might be a relief or a major challenge if your child has been in the hospital for a long time. For many children, going back to school signals a return to normal life. Other children, especially teens, may dread returning to school because of changes in appearance or concerns that prolonged absences may have changed their social standing with their friends.

Most of the information in this chapter deals with schooling for children with a long-term illness or repeated hospitalizations. Educating these children can become complicated, but usually can be managed successfully through planning and good communication.

Keep the school informed

If your child will miss more than a week or two of school, you should notify the school in writing about your child's medical situation. If not notified, schools can drop children from the rolls due to non-attendance. Usually, the school will designate a person (e.g., child's teacher, guidance counselor) to communicate with a designated person at the hospital (e.g., school liaison, child life specialist, social worker). This appointed school liaison will keep information flowing between the hospital and school, and will help pave the way for your child's successful return to class. Because privacy laws prohibit this exchange of information, parents need to sign a release form authorizing the school and hospital to share information. These forms are available at schools and hospitals.

> We had absolutely no problem keeping the school informed as we lived directly behind it. The teacher would frequently stop by on her way home to drop off homework assignments and cards or messages from Stephan's classmates. The school nurse, psychologist, and teacher were at my beck and call. Whenever I felt that we needed to talk, I'd call and they would set up a meeting within twenty-four hours. They have been wonderful.

Keep teachers and classmates involved

If your child is hospitalized for a long time, it helps to stay connected with the teacher and classmates. Parents can help by calling the teacher periodically and bringing notes or taped messages from the sick child to her classmates. Following are some suggestions for keeping the teacher and classmates involved with your child's life:

- Have the nurse or social worker come to class to give a presentation about what is happening to their classmate and how he will look and feel when he returns. This talk should include a question and answer session to clear up misconceptions and alleviate fears. All children, especially teenagers, should be involved in deciding what information should be discussed with classmates and whether or not the child/teen wants to be present.

> We have worked to educate ourselves and our son about his heart problems. Now, if David gets teased at the beginning of the school year, he tells the class exactly what's wrong with his heart. He's very open and truthful about it and they respect him for it. They are nicer after he tells them. They can respect his differences and understand why he is the way he is.

- Encourage classmates to keep in touch by sending notes, calling on the telephone, sending class pictures, or making a banner. (Other ideas are contained in Chapter 11, *Families and Friends: How to Help.*)

- If your child is old enough, allow her to establish a page on a social network site so she can communicate with her friends, express her feelings and thoughts, post photos, and remain connected.

- If possible, use Skype® or a similar webcam software program to allow your child to interact "face-to-face" with classmates on the internet, a smartphone, or another electronic device.

Keeping up with schoolwork

A child who is out of school longer than two weeks for any medical reason is entitled by law to instruction at home or in the hospital. It is a good idea to request off-site instruction as soon as you find out your child may be out of school for longer than two weeks. The school will require a letter from the doctor stating the reason and expected length of time this service will be needed.

Some states require school districts to provide hospital tutoring when children are hospitalized for long stays. Most large children's hospitals have teachers on staff, as well as educational liaisons who can help you work out appropriate schooling.

If your child will miss less than two weeks of school, you can communicate with the teacher to keep abreast of subjects being covered in your child's class. The teacher might send assignments and materials home with siblings, or you can make arrangements for friends or relatives to pick them up.

> We used Skype® and had a weekly time set up so that Mike could see his classmates, and they could see him. If an oral presentation was due, he heard a few of theirs, and presented his. If nothing shareable was due, they just traded jokes or did a show and tell of something that had happened that week. If he was not feeling well or was hospitalized, the call was cancelled for that week. It sure helped make him still feel a part of his class, and the teacher said it really helped his classmates to see he was still okay, and still himself. He wasn't able to attend school at all for almost 10 months.

> Mike started the first day of 5th grade this year. He was able to walk in the building, feel welcome, and step right back into his friendships. No problems at all with that. I really thank his teacher last year for keeping him a part of his class despite not being in school.

Returning to school

The sooner a child can return to school, the better. Preparation and communication are key to a successful return. If your child has only missed a week or two, work with the teacher to find ways for your child to catch up. If, however, your child has been gone for an extended period, ask the physician or primary nurse to prepare a letter for the school staff containing the following information:

- Your child's health status and its probable effect on attendance.

- Whether he can attend regular physical education classes, physical education with restrictions (no running, for example), or adaptive physical education.

> My high-school gym teacher gave me a B after I tore the ligament in my knee and had surgery. Even though I was able to lift weights during class, I couldn't participate in regular class activities. In hindsight, I should have fought this or negotiated to drop the class and take it again later.

- Whether adjustments in your child's schedule are needed. For example, a child with a cast on her arm will be unable to complete a typing class and may benefit from changing classes, even if this isn't standard school procedure.

> My 16-year-old son was allowed to leave each textbook in his various classrooms. This prevented him from having to carry a heavy backpack all day. They also let him out of class a few minutes early, because he was slower moving from room to room.

- A description of any changes in physical appearance, perhaps with suggestions on how to discuss this with classmates.

- The possible effect of medications on academic performance.

- Whether school personnel must administer medications or other services as directed by a doctor.

- Any special considerations such as extra snacks, rest periods, or extra time to get from class to class.

When Brent returned to kindergarten after a long stay in the hospital, he was exhausted. There was a beanbag chair in the back of his classroom, and he just curled up in it and went to sleep when he needed to.

- A list of signs and symptoms requiring parent notification, such as fever, nausea, pain, or swelling.

Stress that the teacher's job is to teach, and the parent and school nurse will take care of all medical issues.

I'm a school nurse. I like parents and their children to come and talk with me when it's time for the child to reenter school. We talk about how the child is feeling, how many hours a day he should be in school, and whether he needs to come rest in my office. I remind parents that I need doctor's orders to give meds or provide nursing services. I love it when parents share information through conversation, journal articles, or brochures. I also prepare the child's class for reentry. I give talks and show videos. I find children to be wonderfully receptive and helpful when they are given truthful information.

Once teachers have had a chance to read the letter, request a meeting that includes the teacher, principal, school nurse, and school counselor or psychologist. At this meeting, answer any questions about the information contained in the letter, distribute any useful information you have, and do your best to establish a rapport with the entire staff. Take this opportunity to express appreciation for the school's help and your hopes for a close collaboration in the future to create a supportive climate for your child.

The following are additional parent suggestions on how to prevent problems through preparation and communication:

- Keep the school informed and involved from the beginning. This fosters a spirit that "we're all in this together."

- If your child has a long-term illness, bring the nurse into the class whenever necessary to talk about your child's illness or injury and answer questions.

- Ask the school to bend some rules and policies if you think it will help your youngster.

- Find ways to check your child's progress after she returns to school. Some children, especially teens, are reluctant to talk about school with parents, but they may need a parent's help negotiating changes in school schedules or rules.

- Volunteer at school if you feel it is important to be nearby in case of problems.

- Realize that teachers and other school staff can be frightened, overwhelmed, and discouraged when they have a child with a serious illness in their classroom. Accurate information and words of appreciation can help immensely.

Siblings and school

Siblings can be overlooked while parents deal with a very ill or hurt child. Many siblings keep their feelings bottled up inside to prevent placing additional burdens on their parents. Often, their stress is most obvious at school. Some parents occasionally allow their healthy siblings to play hooky to be with the ill child in the hospital or to stay at home to rest.

Remember to include the siblings' teachers in all conferences at school. They should be told about the stresses facing the family and understand that feelings may bubble to the surface in their classroom. Encourage school personnel to ask the siblings, "I know your brother is very sick, but how are you doing?"

> Lindsey was in kindergarten when Jesse first got sick. Because we heard nothing from the kindergarten teacher, we assumed that things were going well. At the end of the year, the teacher told us that Lindsey frequently spent part of each day hiding under her desk. When I asked why we had never been told, the teacher said she thought that we already had enough to worry about dealing with Jesse's illness and treatment. She was wrong to make decisions for us, but I wish we had been more attentive. Lindsey needed help.

Chapter 16

Medical and Financial Records

"What the world really needs is
more love and less paperwork."

— Pearl Bailey

KEEPING TRACK OF MEDICAL AND FINANCIAL PAPERWORK can be a trial. For short hospital stays, it involves keeping track of procedures, medications, discharge information, and bills. For longer stays, it can sometimes become overwhelming. But, having easy access to medical reports and a system to organize bills helps save money and decrease stress. This chapter suggests a few simple ways to keep medical and financial records.

Medical records

Think of yourself as someone with two sets of books—the hospital's and your own. If the hospital misplaces lab results, you will still have your copies. If your child's chart becomes a foot thick, you will have a system that makes it easy to spot trends and retrieve dosage information. Even in this age of electronic medical records, doctor's notes and lab results can be misfiled or lost at the hospital.

If you want to keep detailed records, you can record:

- Dates of hospitalizations
- Dates of all medical appointments and the names of the doctors seen
- Dates and results of all lab work
- Dates of treatments, including drugs given and dose
- Side effects from drugs

- Dates and types of any procedures done
- Your child's sleeping patterns, appetite, and emotions

If your child has an emergency illness or injury, you may not be able to keep records as described. Try at least to record what procedures and surgeries occurred, and the names of the doctors involved. This allows you to check your bills for accuracy later.

Parents whose children have been hospitalized suggest many different ways to keep records, including:

- **Journal.** Writing in an electronic or paper notebook works extremely well for people who like to write. Parents make entries every day about all pertinent medical information and often include personal information, such as their feelings or memorable things their child says. Journals are easy to carry back and forth to the hospital, and can be written in while waiting for appointments. One disadvantage is that they can be misplaced, but an advantage is that the journal can be handed off when a spouse or family member is coming to take over hospital duty.

   > I had a paper and pen sitting right there by Chase, and every now and again I picked it up and wrote something in my journal. Some days it was just my thoughts and feelings. Other days I wrote down details of Chase's treatment. Some days I wrote down things like, "Chase is really cranky today," or "He's running a high temperature." I actually had doctors write in my journal if I couldn't spell something or I wanted them to explain the treatment. It really helped.

- **Hospital-supplied charts.** Many hospitals give parents folders containing photocopied sheets for record-keeping.

- **Three-ring binder and hole punch.** A three-ring binder is a handy way to keep copies of lab reports, consent forms, hospital admission forms, discharge orders, and other hospital paperwork all in one place.

   > Record-keeping—very important! My father came to the hospital soon after diagnosis and brought a three-ring binder

*and a three-hole punch. I would punch lab reports, protocols,
consent forms, drug information sheets, etc., and keep them in
my binder.*

- **Computer or tablet (e.g., iPad® or Surface®).** For many families, keeping all medical and financial records on a laptop or tablet is an attractive option.

Your records will help you remember questions, prevent mistakes, and notice trends.

Financial records

Even when you have good insurance and your child's hospital stay is short, it pays to keep good records, stay alert for billing inaccuracies, and get problems resolved quickly. These days, the cost for short stays or simple procedures can quickly reach very large amounts. In addition, many expenditures that you pay out of pocket may be deductible on your federal tax return. Knowing what expenses are tax-deductible will help you keep the necessary records now and possibly save money at tax time.

For most financial records, you will need just an expandable folder. If your child's illness involves many or lengthy hospitalizations, you will probably need a well-organized file cabinet. Here are a few suggestions for ways to manage your financial records:

- Set up a folder system or files just for medical expense records, such as hospital bills, doctor bills, all other medical bills, insurance explanations of benefits (EOBs), prescription receipts, and correspondence.

- Whenever you open an envelope containing medical billing or insurance information, file the contents immediately. Don't put it on a pile or throw it in a drawer.

- Keep a notebook with a running log of all tax-deductible medical expenses, including the service, charge, bill paid, date paid, and check number.

Deductible medical expenses

The Internal Revenue Service (IRS) generally allows you to deduct any reasonable cost for procedures or expenses that are deemed by a doctor to be medically necessary. You may also deduct other expenses with proper documentation, such as meals, parking, transportation to and from the hospital or doctor's appointments, lodging costs while your child is in the hospital, wheelchairs, acupuncture, and insurance premiums for medical coverage.

To find out what can be deducted, get IRS Publication 502 for the relevant tax year. You can download this publication from the IRS website at *www.irs.gov* or make a copy from a hard-copy master at your local public library. You can contact an IRS representative at (800) 829-1040, Monday through Friday.

Problems with hospital bills

Not everyone experiences billing problems. People who have managed health care plans or who receive public assistance may never see bills. Some families have no problems with bills from the hospital. But many parents of children who spend time in the hospital encounter billing problems. Although it is impossible to prevent billing errors, it is necessary to deal with them. Here are step-by-step suggestions for solving billing problems:

- Check every bill from the hospital to make sure there are no charges for treatments not given or for errors, such as double billing.

    I go through every bill looking for errors. When David had angioplasty and catheterization, the hospital part of the bill came to twenty thousand dollars. By the time I was done with the bill, it was only nine thousand dollars because I found so many errors.

- Contact a financial counselor at the hospital if you have any problems with billing. Financial counselors can help you understand the hospital's billing system, work out a payment plan, and resolve disputes.

- Don't pay a bill unless you have checked each item to make sure the charge is correct.

- Compare each hospital bill to the explanation of benefits (EOBs) you receive from your insurance company and investigate any discrepancies.

    Our insurance paid 80 percent of everything, no questions asked, and always paid within a month. We never had a problem. People shouldn't have to worry about finances or their insurance program at a difficult time like this.

- Call the billing department of the hospital immediately if you find a error. Write down the date, the name of the person you talk to, and the plan of action.

- If the error is not corrected on your next bill, call and talk to the billing supervisor. Explain politely the steps you have already taken and how you would like the problem fixed.

    The hospital billing was so bad, and I had to call so often, that I developed a telephone relationship with the billing supervisor. I always tried to be upbeat, we laughed a lot, and it worked out. She stopped investigating every problem and would just delete the erroneous charge.

- Ask a family member or friend to help if you are too tired or overwhelmed to deal with the bills. Your friend could come every other week, open and file all bills and insurance papers, make phone calls, and write all necessary letters.

- Don't let billing problems accumulate. Your account may end up at a collection agency, which can quickly become a huge headache.

    Within five months of my daughter's diagnosis, the billing was so messed up that I despaired of ever getting it straight. When the hospital threatened to send the account to a collection agency, I took action. I wrote letters to the hospital and the insurance company demanding that they each audit our account. When both audits arrived, they were thousands of dollars apart. I met with our insurance representative. She called the hospital, and we had a three-way conversation. We straightened it out that time, but every bill that I received had one or more errors, always in the hospital's favor.

Chapter 17

Insurance

"Be it better or be it worse
Please you the man that bears the purse."

— Thomas Delaney

FINDING ONE'S WAY THROUGH THE INSURANCE MAZE can be a difficult task. However, understanding the benefits and claims procedures can help you get the bills paid without undue stress. This chapter describes some steps to help prevent problems with insurance.

Understand your policy

As soon as you know a hospitalization is necessary, it helps to read your entire insurance manual and make a list of any questions you have about terms or benefits. The human resources department at your workplace can answer questions about your policy or direct you to someone who can.

- Learn who the "participating providers" are under the plan and what happens if you see a "non-participating provider." You may have to pay more or your claims may be denied if you go to a doctor or hospital that does not have a contract with your insurance company—this is called going "outside the network."

- Find out when you have to precertify a hospitalization. Many insurance companies require precertification, even for emergencies.

> I realized that Christine had been hospitalized for a week,
> and I had not called the insurance company. When I read the
> manual, I was upset to find out that there was a two hundred
> dollar penalty for not calling them, even though it was an emer-
> gency admission.

- Find out when a second opinion is required.

- Determine whether your doctor needs to document specific requirements to obtain coverage for expensive or extended services.

   With our insurance, occupational therapy, speech therapy, and physical therapy are covered, but the phrasing in the doctor's orders must be that each service is a "medical necessity."

- Find out what your deductible is.

- Find out if there is a point at which coverage increases to 100 percent.

Find a case manager

If your child has a long-term illness or an injury that requires many hospitalizations, call your insurance company and ask who will handle your claims. Explain the situation to your insurance representative and tell her it would be helpful to always deal with the same person. Insurers sometimes will assign a case manager to review claims, handle special needs, and answer any questions that you have about benefits. Try to develop a cooperative relationship with your case manager because he can make your life much easier. Your employer may also have a benefits specialist who can serve as a liaison with the insurer.

Don't be afraid to negotiate benefits with the insurance company. Your case manager may be able to redefine a service that your child needs so it will be covered.

   Our insurance company covered 100 percent of "maintenance drugs" only if the patient needed them for the rest of their lives. Katy's drugs were only needed for two years but were extremely expensive. I asked my contact person for help, and she petitioned the decision-making board. They granted us an exemption and covered the entire cost of all her medication for two years.

The key to obtaining the maximum benefit from your insurance policy is to keep accurate records and appeal any denied claims, sometimes more than once. Some tips for good record-keeping follow:

- Keep accurate records of all medical expenses and claims submitted.

- Write down the date, name of person contacted, and content of all phone calls about insurance.

- Make photocopies of anything you send to your insurance company, including appeal letters.

- Pay bills by check or credit card, and keep all your canceled checks and/or credit card monthly summaries of charges.

- Keep all correspondence you receive from billing companies and insurance.

Appealing a denial

If any of your insurance claims are denied, you have the right to appeal the decision and have it reviewed by a third party. First, make sure that the service is covered by your insurance policy. If it is, following are suggested steps to appeal the denial:

- Read your policy or the back of the explanation of benefits to learn what your insurance company's appeals procedures are. Sometimes there is a time limit, so you need to file the written appeal before your time runs out.

- No matter what they tell you on the phone, appeals must be filed in writing.

- Write a clear letter explaining why the insurance company should reconsider its decision, and attach a copy of the denial letter from the insurance company. Keep original documents in your files. Insurance companies have to respond in writing to your written appeal to explain why they denied your claim (this is called an "internal review").

- If your claim is denied a second time, request an "external review." In this process, your appeal will go to an independent third party for review.

- If you have problems with the appeal process, you can contact your elected representative to the U.S. Congress. All Senators and members of the House of Representatives have staff members who help constituents with problems.

- You can also contact your state insurance commission with concerns and complaints.

> When I ran into insurance company problems, I wrote a letter to the insurance company detailing the facts, the decisions the insurance company made, and a logical explanation about why the procedure needed to happen. I also noted on the letter that a copy was going to our state insurance commissioner, and I sent both letters by certified mail. Within two days, the insurance company all of a sudden decided to cover the procedure. I later found out that the insurance commissioner's office started an investigation against the company. Letters help, especially when sent by certified mail.

You may not feel comfortable being so persistent, but sometimes it is necessary to ensure you get the coverage you and your child are legally entitled to receive.

> When I finally got a case manager assigned for my child within our insurance company, I fretted to her one day that every single claim was initially rejected. She replied that the agents were trained to reject all claims the first two times they were submitted as a cost-saving strategy. She said, "Very few subscribers are tenacious enough to come back three times, so we save millions of dollars each year just because they give up."

Staying insured

Loss of insurance coverage is a huge worry for many parents. If you lose your job, change jobs, or move while your child is ill, speak to your employer's benefits manager promptly. You can continue insurance coverage with your previous employer through the Consolidated Omnibus Budget Reconciliation Act (COBRA) plan until you are certain your new insurance coverage is in effect or you can look for coverage under the Affordable Care Act (*www. healthfinder.gov*).

> *We just switched to an ACA [Affordable Care Act] plan from COBRA, as did a friend of mine with cancer. I am saving $300 per month and she is saving $400. ACA covers preexisting conditions, and you can get a special tax credit that is not available with COBRA if your income level is within certain limits.*

Chapter 18

Sources of Financial Help

"Lack of money is trouble without equal."
— Rabelais

SOURCES OF FINANCIAL ASSISTANCE VARY from state to state and town to town. To track down possible sources, you can ask the hospital social worker or a social worker at your local health department for help. Some hospitals also have community outreach nurses or case workers who may point out helpful resources.

Hospital policy

If you are unable to pay your hospital bills, don't let your account go to a collection agency or take out a large loan to pay the bill. Make an appointment with a hospital financial counselor to discuss the hospital's financial assistance policy. Many hospitals write off a percentage of the cost of care if the patient is uninsured or underinsured. You may also be able to set up a payment plan based on your income.

Supplemental Security Income

SSI is an entitlement program of the federal government that is based on family income and administered by the Social Security Administration. Recipients must be blind or disabled and have a low family income and few assets. If you think your child might qualify for SSI, contact your nearest field office.

In addition, if you need legal help appealing a denial for SSI, there is a professional organization of attorneys and paralegals called the National Organization for Social Security Claimants' Representatives

(NOSSCR). NOSSCR can refer you to a member in your geographic location. You can contact NOSSCR by phone at (800) 431-2804, or online at *www.nosscr.org*.

State-sponsored supplemental insurance

Most states have supplemental insurance programs for families with children who are living with chronic conditions. These programs often help cover services, prescriptions, and copayments that your primary insurance will not. You can get more information about the specific programs in your state from your hospital social worker, or by calling your state's department that regulates insurance (e.g., State Insurance Commission).

> *In Michigan, besides my husband's insurance, we also have what is called Children's Special Health Care Services (CSHCS). It is a secondary insurance that pays for what our primary insurance doesn't: co-pays and prescriptions, trips back and forth to the hospital, doctor appointment and prescription co-pays for my husband and me, our stay at the Ronald McDonald House. Any expenses related to treatment that our primary insurance won't cover, this will. The amount you pay for this coverage is based on family income. It has been a lifesaver for us.*

Medicaid

Medicaid is administered by state governments in the United States, with the federal government providing a portion of the cost. Rules about eligibility vary, but families with private insurance are sometimes eligible if huge hospital bills are only partially covered. Call your local or county social service department to obtain the number for the Medicaid office in your area. Medicaid sometimes pays transportation and prescription costs. Some states cover children under the age of 21 if they are hospitalized for more than 30 continuous days, regardless of parental income. A hospital social worker or financial counselor can help you determine if your family is eligible for benefits.

Free medicine programs

Children sometimes need expensive medications that insurance will not cover. Most major U.S. drug companies have patient-assistance programs, and you can apply to obtain free or low-cost prescription drugs. Although each company has its own criteria for qualification, in general, you must:

• Be a U.S. citizen or legal resident

• Have a prescription for the medication you are applying to get

• Have no prescription drug coverage for the medication

• Meet income requirements

You may qualify even if you have health insurance, if it does not cover the medication prescribed to your child. For expensive medications, the income cut-off is high, so it is worth investigating whether or not you qualify. Several organizations that can help you find and apply to patient-assistance programs are listed in *Resources*. Because the application process takes time and includes obtaining information from your child's doctor(s), plan ahead so you do not run out of medication.

> *Our insurance does not cover the growth hormone that my daughter needs. Her physician cannot believe that our insurance company denied coverage given her medical history, but that's our situation. The medication is incredibly expensive. We applied to a patient-assistance program and were thrilled to find out that we qualified if our adjusted gross income was less than $100,000 a year. The application process the first year was hard and took a few months, but now we just fill in a form and send in our tax return every year, and she is requalified. We get a shipment of growth hormone every three months and keep it in the fridge.*

Service organizations

Many service organizations help families in need. They can provide transportation, special equipment, or food. Often, all a family has to do is describe their plight, and good Samaritans appear. Some organizations that may have chapters in your community are: American

Legion; Elks Club; fraternal organizations such as Masons, Jaycees, Kiwanis Club, Knights of Columbus, Lions, Rotary; United Way; Veterans of Foreign Wars; and religious organizations of all denominations. Local philanthropic organizations also help needy families in many communities. To find them, call your local health department, speak to the social worker, and ask for help. In addition to local organizations, numerous programs fly children free of charge to the best hospital for their medical needs. The *Resources* section of the book contains contact information for several of these organizations.

Organized fundraising

Many communities rally around a sick or injured child by organizing a fundraiser. Help is given in various ways, ranging from donation jars in local stores to an organized fund drive using all the local media. There are many pitfalls to avoid in fund raising, and great care must be exercised to protect the child's privacy as much as possible. Because there have been some unfortunate scams in which generous people were bilked out of contributions for sick children who did not exist, if you decide to try fundraising, it is best to obtain legal assistance so donations will go into a trust fund to pay your child's medical expenses.

If your child is on or seeking SSI or Medicaid eligibility, donated funds must be held in a special needs trust and paid directly to providers. If the family receives the money, or the child's Social Security number is used to open the bank account, the child can lose funding from both SSI and Medicaid.

Chapter 19

Looking Back

"Time cools, time clarifies."
— Thomas Mann

HOSPITAL STAYS CAN BE physically and emotionally challenging for children, siblings, parents, family, and friends. However, facing and dealing with adversity causes change and, often, growth. The dozens of parents who shared their stories in this book described many benefits and positive aftereffects for all members of the family.

Children who have short stays or outpatient procedures, reported learning about:

- How their body works
- The type of work that doctors and nurses do
- The types of medical problems that other children face
- How to manage a difficult or painful experience

The lives of families of children who endure long or frequent hospitalizations are often changed forever. Although acknowledging the challenges, parents, children, and siblings also described many longlasting benefits from their experiences.

- **Appreciation.** Looking back, many parents reflected on the people they met. They describe kids with incredible courage, parents they will never forget, and caregivers who just never stopped giving. The people they met in hospitals whose situations were very grave bestowed a renewed appreciation for life. Many parents said they now cherish the little things: their child's smile, the first hug of the day, the morning sun. Life slows down, and is savored.

- **Awareness.** Parents described the incredible intensity of their child's hospital experience. One mother said, "So much happened so quickly, and was so emotionally powerful, that we felt like we were in a true life drama unfolding in the hospital room." The emotions experienced by children and parents alike changed their awareness of normal. Life seemed fuller and richer than in the past.

- **Bonding.** Sharing a hospital experience, day and night, with your child can forge close bonds. It gives parents and child time together, to talk, to play, to cry, and sometimes to laugh. Children realize the enormity of their parent's love, and parents often become closer to their child simply by sharing these experiences.

- **Emotions.** Parents shared that the experience of living through a serious illness and hospitalization brought their emotions closer to the surface. They cry more and they laugh louder. They learned to make every day count and to weave wonderful memories out of little things the family shared. Hugs became valuable, and, many years later, they still hug each other more. They learned to reach out and show people how much they care.

- **Knowledge of the medical system.** Any involvement with the medical system increases parents' and children's knowledge. Parents who are involved over long periods of time become masters at working the system effectively. Often, they become advocates for friends or relatives who call for advice or support. They are no longer intimidated by the hospital, they understand why and how things work, and they often use this knowledge to help others.

- **Knowledge about illness and injuries.** Both children and parents learn a great deal about illness, kindness, and ways to help people who are hurting. They develop true compassion from their experiences in the hospital and the friends they made there. Many children who have endured long hospitalizations, as well as their siblings, plan careers in the helping professions. It can transform their lives.

- **Confidence.** The confidence of "having been there, done that" hones children's and parents' abilities to help others in crisis. They know just the right things to say and do when a friend is in the hospital. They are comfortable visiting the hospital, talking to doctors, offering help, and exploring treatment options. Their medical competence is high.

❧

The parents who contributed to this book hope that your child's hospitalization enriched all of your lives in unexpected ways, and that your future is full of good health and happiness.

My Hospital Journal

My name: _____

_____

Date I came to the hospital: _____

_____

Name of the hospital: _____

_____

_____

Before I came to the hospital

What I thought it would be like: _____

_____

_____

_____

_____

What my parents told me: _____

_____

_____

_____

What the hospital tour was like: _____

_____

_____

_____

What I packed: _____

_____

_____

_____

_____

My room

My room number: _____

My bed: _____

What I see out my window: _____

_____

_____

_____

_____

How I decorate my room: _____

_____

_____

_____

_____

_____

_____

_____

_____

Why I am in the hospital

*How my parents describe it:*_____

_____

_____

_____

_____

*How my doctor describes it:*_____

_____

_____

_____

_____

What I think of it: _____

_____

_____

_____

_____

_____

_____

_____

_____

My doctor(s)

My doctor's name: _____

_____

What I call him/her: _____

_____

What I like best about my doctor: _____

_____

_____

_____

My doctor writes a note: _____

_____

_____

_____

_____

_____

_____

_____

_____

My nurses

My nurses' names: _____

_____

_____

What I call them: _____

_____

_____

What I like best about my nurses: _____

_____

_____

_____

My nurses write a note: _____

_____

_____

_____

_____

_____

_____

My roommate(s)

My roommate's name: _____
_____

Why my roommate is in the hospital: _____
_____
_____

Where my roommate lives: _____
_____

What I like about sharing a room: _____
_____
_____
_____

What I don't like: _____
_____
_____
_____
_____
_____

My school

My teacher's name: _____

_____

_____

My best friends at school: _____

_____

_____

_____

How my class will know I am in the hospital: _____

_____

_____

How many days of school I am missing: _____

_____

How I do my homework: _____

_____

_____

_____

_____

People who sent me cards or gifts

_____

_____

_____

_____

_____

_____

_____

_____

_____

_____

_____

_____

_____

_____

_____

_____

_____

Friends' sign-in sheet

_____

_____

_____

_____

_____

_____

_____

_____

_____

_____

_____

_____

_____

_____

_____

_____

_____

Relatives' sign-in sheet

_____

_____

_____

_____

_____

_____

_____

_____

_____

_____

_____

_____

_____

_____

_____

_____

Meals in the hospital

What I order for meals: _____

_____

_____

Favorite breakfast: _____

_____

Favorite lunch: _____

_____

Favorite dinner: _____

_____

Hospital food I don't like: _____

_____

Food I can't have: _____

_____

_____

_____

_____

Places I've been to in the hospital

_____ *Lobby*

_____ *Gift shop*

_____ *Cafeteria*

_____ *Playroom*

_____ *Elevator*

_____ *Operating room*

_____ *Recovery room*

_____ *Nurses' station*

_____ *X-ray room*

Others: _____

_____

_____

_____

_____

_____

_____

_____

What happens at night in the hospital

What it sounds like: _____

_____

_____

_____

When the nurses come in: _____

_____

_____

_____

What nurses do at night: _____

_____

_____

_____

What I like: _____

_____

What I don't like: _____

_____

What I miss from home

My brother(s): _____

_____

_____

My sister(s): _____

_____

_____

My pets: _____

_____

My friends: _____

_____

My bed: _____

What else? _____

_____

_____

_____

_____

Playing in the hospital

How I play in my room: _____

_____

_____

What the hospital playroom is like: _____

_____

_____

How I go to the playroom: _____

_____

Who helps kids in the playroom: _____

_____

What toys are there: _____

_____

Other kids I met in the playroom: _____

_____

_____

_____

Medicine

Pills I have to take: _____
_____
_____

How the pills taste: _____
_____
_____

Liquid medicine I have to take: _____
_____
_____

How my liquid medicine tastes: _____
_____
_____

How often I have medicine: _____
_____

How I feel about my medicines: _____
_____

Tests in the hospital

_____ CAT scan

_____ X-ray

_____ Blood draw

Others: _____

_____

Tests I like the best: _____

_____

_____

_____

Tests I don't like: _____

_____

_____

_____

Prizes I get: _____

_____

_____

_____

Operation

What my operation is for: _____

_____

_____

_____

What my bandages look like: _____

_____

_____

_____

My surgeon's name: _____

_____

What I remember: _____

_____

_____

_____

_____

_____

_____

_____

Going home

How long I stayed in the hospital: _____

_____

_____

The day I left the hospital: _____

_____

How I went from my room to the front door of the hospital:

_____

_____

What it was like outside: _____

_____

_____

Who drove me home: _____

_____

How I felt about leaving: _____

_____

_____

Memories

What I remember most: _____

_____

_____

_____

_____

_____

_____

_____

How I'll feel if I have to go to the hospital again: _____

_____

_____

_____

_____

_____

_____

Packing List

Clothing

___ shirts

___ pants

___ underwear

___ pajamas

___ bathrobe

___ slippers

___ shoes

___ socks

For the room

___ blankets

___ bedspread/quilt

___ comfy pillow

___ pictures of family, friends, pets

___ posters

___ tape to put up pictures and posters

___ balloons/streamers/crepe paper

___ books and magazines

___ laptap or tablet

___ cell phone and charger

___ snack foods and drinks

___ flashlight

Toys

___ stuffed animals

___ dolls

___ children's books

___ playing cards

___ board games

___ puzzles

___ puppets

___ craft projects

___ computer games

___ music

___ extra batteries or chargers

___ squirt gun

___ pens, pencils, paper

___ art materials: markers, paints, crayons

___ joke book

Hygiene

___ eyeglasses

___ toothbrush

___ toothpaste

___ dental floss

___ tissues

___ body lotion

Hygiene (cont.)

___ shampoo/conditioner

___ soap

___ brush/comb

___ nail clippers

___ earplugs

Miscellaneous

___ camera

___ money

___ sewing kit

___ safety pins

___ hot water bottle

Resources

Books for children

Alex and the Amazing Lemonade Stand
Jay and Liz Scott, 2004

Using rhymes and whimsical pictures, this inspirational book tells the true story of a little girl who decided to help fund medical research by opening a lemonade stand. It shows how the small act of one child can inspire thousands of people.

Busy World of Richard Scarry: A Big Operation
Richard Scarry, 1995

In this charming story, Huckle has to have his tonsils out and is a little afraid of the hospital. Lowly takes him around the hospital so he can see and talk to other people who have had operations, and Huckle isn't scared anymore.

Clifford Visits the Hospital
Norman Bridwell, 2012

Clifford visits the hospital and gets into mischief everywhere he goes.

Cooper Gets a Cast
Karen Olson, 2003

Cooper falls out of his tree house and hurts his leg. His dad takes him to the hospital and a nice nurse helps get his leg ready for an x-ray. The doctor shows Cooper his broken bone on the x-ray film and tells him he needs a cast. Cooper goes home and tells his dog, Bunker, about the experience.

Curious George Goes to the Hospital
Margaret and H. A. Rey, 2008

George swallows a piece of a puzzle and must be taken to the hospital for an operation. Through his eyes (and the colorful illustrations), children get a sense of the hospital experience and enjoy a happy ending when a healthy George returns home with his friend.

Don't You Feel Well, Sam?
Amy Hest, 2007

A gentle, beautifully illustrated book about Sam taking his medicine.

Franklin Goes to the Hospital
Sharon Jennings, 2011

Franklin goes to the hospital for an operation to repair his broken shell, and everyone thinks he's being very brave. But Franklin is only pretending to be fearless. He's worried that his x-rays will show just how frightened he is inside. With the help of Dr. Bear, Franklin learns that even though he's feeling scared, he can still be brave.

Going to the Hospital
Fred Rogers, 1997

In his usual tone of sympathetic understanding and gentle reassurance, Mr. Rogers follows two preschool age children, a pigtailed black girl and red-headed white boy, as they experience getting an identification bracelet, being examined with various instruments, having blood drawn, and talking with a nurse and doctor.

Good-bye Tonsils!
Craig and Juliana Hatkoff, 2004

Dr. Ward and Juliana's parents help Juliana understand what will happen when she's in the hospital. By the time she has her surgery, she knows just what to expect.

Harry Goes to the Hospital: A Story for Children About What It's Like to Be in the Hospital

Howard Bennett, 2008

When Harry gets stomach flu, he is admitted to the hospital, examined, and given an IV and a lot of tests. The procedures are explained in straightforward language, and Harry's mother remains at his side throughout his stay in the hospital.

Ish

Peter Reynolds, 2004

A wonderful book about creativity and art that will inspire any child in the hospital to draw, write, color, and create, and feel good about himself or herself while doing it.

Little Critter: My Trip to the Hospital

Mercer Mayer, 2012

When Little Critter breaks his leg in a soccer game, he has to make his first trip to the hospital. The book follows Little Critter as he rides in an ambulance, meets the doctor, and gets his first x-ray and his first cast.

Press Here

Herve Tullet, 2011

A charming, interactive book for preschoolers that will take their mind off the hospital and result in many giggles and demands to "Let's do it again!"

This is a Hospital, Not a Zoo!

Roberta Karim, 2002

Filbert MacFee is having a lively time in the hospital. When Nurse Skeeter is ready to give him a shot, he turns into a thick-skinned rhinoceros! The moment he sits in an ice-cold wheelchair headed for x-ray, he becomes a penguin. Crafty Nurse Beluga outwits Filbert in all his animal transformations, but good news comes at last from Dr. Kebob. Once he stops being an orangutan, he tells Filbert he is well enough to go home.

The Surgery Book for Kids
Shivani Bhatia, 2010

Iggy finds out that his snoring and sore throats are caused by his marshmallow-like tonsils, and that he needs surgery. His fears are lessened by learning about the surgery, and his experience turns into an adventure.

A Visit to the Sesame Street Hospital
Deborah Hautzig, 1985

Grover, his mother, Ernie, and Bert visit the Sesame Street Hospital to prepare for Grover's upcoming tonsillectomy. The familiar characters change an unfamiliar hospital into a place to be trusted, and many typical questions are discussed.

Books for parents

Penny Whistle Sick-in-Bed Book: What to Do With Kids When They're Home for a Day, a Week, a Month, or More
Meredith Brokaw, Annie Gilbar, Jill Weber, 1993

Whether your preschooler is home with the chicken pox, or your fifth-grader is laid up with a broken leg, this book comes to the rescue with a delightful collection of absorbing activities to occupy young patients, and advice and ideas for their parents, from setting up a sickroom to helping a bedridden child stay physically fit.

The "O, MY" in Tonsillectomy & Adenoidectomy: How to Prepare Your Child for Surgery, 2nd Edition
Laurie Zelinger, 2010

This book helps parents understand the medical and emotional aspects of their child's surgery. In an easy-to-follow timeline for events before and after a tonsillectomy or adenoidectomy, it provides reassuring and accurate guidance that eases the process for the child and family.

Books for siblings

Becky's Story

Donna Baznik, 1981

Becky is a 6-year-old girl whose brother Dan is seriously injured in an accident. Becky expresses all her turbulent feelings during her brother's hospital stay and talks about how her parents help her through it.

Hi, My Name Is Jack

Christina Beall-Sullivan, 2000

This book is about Jack, the healthy sibling of Molly who has a chronic illness and needs to go to the hospital often. Jack sometimes feels scared and jealous and then angry and guilty about Molly. He wishes his parents had more time for him. When he feels this way, he finds that if he talks to Molly or his parents he feels better. His parents reassure him that Molly's illness is not his fault.

My Brother Needs an Operation

Anna Marie Jaworski, 1998

This book tells the story of a big brother whose younger sibling needs an operation. He faces many emotions, stresses, and worries. The book offers tips for parents to help children cope with their concerns, and includes games and activities that help keep unhospitalized children amused and involved in family life.

When Molly Was in the Hospital: A Book for Brothers and Sisters of Hospitalized Children

Debbie Duncan, 1994

Anna's little sister, Molly, has been very ill and had to have an operation. Anna tells readers about the experience from her point of view in this sensitive, insightful, and heartwarming story.

What About Me? When Brothers and Sisters Get Sick

Alan Peterkin, 1992

When a child is seriously ill, siblings experience mixed emotions and hurt feelings, and wonder about the future. In this heartwarming story, the narrator, a young girl, expresses all of these concerns when her brother goes to the hospital for an extended stay.

Free air travel

Air Charity Network
(877) 621-7177
http://aircharitynetwork.org

Made up of independent member organizations, in specific geographical service areas, that coordinate free airline tickets or reduced-price ambulatory services.

Air Care Alliance
(888) 260-9707
www.aircarealliance.org

Nationwide association of humanitarian flying organizations that provide flights for medical treatment.

Angel Flight
(918) 749-8992
www.angelflight.com

Provides free transportation to medical treatment for people who cannot afford public transportation or who cannot tolerate it for health reasons.

Corporate Angel Network, Inc.
(866) 328-1313
www.corpangelnetwork.org

Gives patients with cancer available seats on corporate aircraft to get to and from recognized cancer treatment centers. Patients must be able to walk and travel without life-support systems or medical attention. A child may be accompanied by up to two adults. Eligibility is not based on financial need.

Miracle Flights for Kids
(800) FLY-1711 / (800) 359-1711
www.miracleflights.org

Helps families overcome financial obstacles by flying their seriously ill children to receive proper medical care and to get second opinions.

Help with insurance

Patient Advocate Foundation (PAF)
(800) 532-5274
www.patientadvocate.org

Provides patients with arbitration, mediation, and negotiation to settle issues with access to care, medical debt, and job retention related to illness.

Medications (low-cost or free)

Partnership for Prescription Assistance
(888) 477-2669
www.pparx.org

Helps find companies and agencies that provide prescription medicines free of charge to physicians whose patients might not otherwise have access to necessary medicines.

RxHope
(877) 267-0517
www.rxhope.com

Lists patient-assistance programs that are offered by federal, state, and charitable organizations.

PatientAssistance.com, Inc.
www.patientassistance.com

Helps uninsured patients get free medication.

NeedyMeds, Inc.
www.needymeds.org

Helps people who cannot afford medicine or healthcare costs. The information at NeedyMeds is available anonymously and free of charge.

Place to stay near hospitals

Ronald McDonald Houses
www.rmhc.com

Provides free or low-cost housing close to hospitals in many major cities for ill children and their families.

Contributors

Brenda Andrews, L. S. Auth, Jodie Barbour, Robin B., Sue Brooks, Edie Cardwell, Carolyn J. Casey, Alicia Cauley, Wendy Corder Dowhower, Debra Ethier, S. Farringer, Lisa Hall, Connie Higbee-Jones, Chris Hurley, Missy Layfield, Deirdre McCarthy-King, Sara McDonnall, Wendy Mitchell, Amanda Moodie, Ann Newman, Robin Aspman-O'Callahan, Christina O'Reilly, Carrie Beth Parigrew, M. Clare Paris, Sandra L. Pilant, Mary C. Riecke, Jennifer M. Rohloff, Sheila Sandiford, Carol Schuette, Mark Schumann, Brenna Scoville, Scott and Richelle Shields, Cathi Poer Smith, Carl and Diane Snedeker, Ralene Walls, Emily Weiner, Kimbra Suzanne Wilder, Jean Wilkinson, Catherine Woodman, Ellen Zimmerman, and those who wish to remain anonymous.

About the Author

Nancy Keene, a well-known writer and advocate for hospitalized children, has written and co-authored twelve consumer health books on topics ranging from childhood illnesses to working with your doctor. Her work has appeared in many publications, including *Reader's Digest, Journal of the American Medical Association, Exceptional Parent,* and *Coping Magazine.* She served as chair of the patient advocacy committee of a consortium of 350 children's hospitals and on a U.S. Food and Drug Administration (FDA) committee that reviewed medications given to ill children. Ms. Keene has been interviewed on National Public Radio (NPR), frequently speaks to professional and parent groups, and has participated in online support groups for parents of ill children since 1996.

About the Publisher

Childhood Cancer Guides, a 501(c)(3) nonprofit, publishes books that help families with ill children. Since 2003, we have been a leading source of understandable and medically reviewed information woven with stories and advice from hundreds of parents, ill children, and their siblings. Our books—a blend of medical information, practical suggestions, and emotional support—help families find a path through medical crises, one step at a time. Visit us at *www.childhoodcancerguides.org*.

Colophon

The cover of *Your Child in the Hospital: A Practical Guide for Parents, Third Edition*, was designed by Michele Keen of Creative Freedom (*www.creativefreedom.com*) and implemented by Susan Jarmolowski, using Adobe Photoshop 12, Illustrator 15, and InDesign 7.5. The cover photo is © Graham Bell/Corbis, and is used with permission.

The interior layout was designed and implemented by Susan Jarmolowski using Adobe InDesign 7.5. This book was edited by Judy Kleinberg (*kleinbergwrites@gmail.com*) and proofread by Alison Leake. Nancy Keene conducted quality checks.